Date: 6/1/20

355.0092 FIG
Fighting with pride : LGBTQ
in the armed forces /

FIGHTING WITH
PRIDE

'*Fighting with Pride* is a captivating book chronicling an incredible period of positive change in the social history of the Armed Forces, told by the women and men whose courage on the battlefield was matched by their courage of conviction. You will be moved by their unstinting loyalty to their Service and Country, with recollections that will make you laugh and shake your head in dismay and disbelief.'

General Sir James Everard KCB CBE, Deputy Supreme
Allied Commander Europe

'This important book records a turning point in LGBT+ equality in the UK and the beginning and end of a remarkable journey for our Armed Forces. Resolute and determined, these are the stories of those whose journeys epitomise what was lost by excluding and what we have gained in equality.'

Baroness Ruth Hunt, Chief Executive of Stonewall, 2014–2019

'These are inspiring personal stories of how LGBT+ service personnel challenged and overturned exclusion and discrimination in the military. They remind us that LGBTs in the Armed Forces were once tasked with defending freedoms that they were themselves denied. But thanks to their resilience, they are at last free and equal. Bravo!'

Peter Tatchell, Human Rights Campaigner and Director of the
Peter Tatchell Foundation

FIGHTING WITH
PRIDE
LGBTQ IN THE ARMED FORCES

EDITED BY
CRAIG JONES

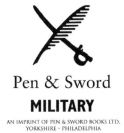

Pen & Sword
MILITARY

AN IMPRINT OF PEN & SWORD BOOKS LTD.
YORKSHIRE - PHILADELPHIA

First published in Great Britain in 2019 by
PEN & SWORD MILITARY
An imprint of
Pen & Sword Books Ltd
Yorkshire - Philadelphia

ISBN 978 1 52676 525 3

Typeset in Ehrhardt MT & 11/13
by Aura Technology and Software Services, India

Printed and bound in England by TJ International Ltd.

Pen & Sword Books Ltd incorporates the Imprints of Pen & Sword Archaeology,
Atlas, Aviation, Battleground, Discovery, Family History, History, Maritime,
Military, Naval, Politics, Railways, Select, Transport, True Crime, Fiction,
Frontline Books, Leo Cooper, Praetorian Press, Seaforth Publishing, Wharncliffe
and White Owl.

For a complete list of Pen & Sword titles please contact

PEN & SWORD BOOKS LIMITED
47 Church Street, Barnsley, South Yorkshire, S70 2AS, England
E-mail: enquiries@pen-and-sword.co.uk
Website: www.pen-and-sword.co.uk

Or

PEN AND SWORD BOOKS
1950 Lawrence Rd, Havertown, PA 19083, USA
E-mail: uspen-and-sword@casematepublishers.com
Website: www.penandswordbooks.com

This book is dedicated to those dismissed, retired and serving who have been proud to serve and who now serve with pride.

'When I was in the military they gave me a medal for killing
two men and a discharge for loving one.'

Sergeant Leonard Philip Matlovich (6 July 1943 – 22 June 1988),
Vietnam War veteran and recipient of the
Purple Heart and Bronze Star

'Those who can imagine anything, can create the impossible.'

Alan Turing OBE FRS, Leader of Hut 8 at Bletchley Park,
where the Enigma code was broken

Contents

Acknowledgements

The authors wish to express their appreciation to:

Robert Ely, who, with Elaine Chambers, co-founded Rank Outsiders, an organisation that picked up the banner of the military covenant as it fell to the ground.

The Armed Forces Legal Challenge Group, founded by Ed Hall, and also to Lord David Pannick QC for winning a case that was the first crack in the wall of LGBTQ inequality.

Lord Michael Cashman CBE, Founding Chair of Stonewall, and Angela Mason CBE, Chief Executive of Stonewall 1992–2002, for supporting the legal campaign amidst a mix of priorities.

Associate Professor Aaron Belkin of the Palm Centre at the University of California for his twenty-five years of support of the UK and US Armed Forces communities.

Squadron Leader Philip Johnston-Davis RAF and Nick Johnston-Davis, founders of Proud2Serve, which helped bring us all together in the years after the ban was lifted.

Ian Romanis, of the Civil Service LGBT Forum, for his support within the MoD Civil Service.

Admiral Lord West of Spithead GCB, DSC, PC, for his support as First Sea Lord and Chief of the Naval Staff.

Lady 'Rosie' West for sprinkling fairy dust on the pathway of progress.

The Royal Navy Chaplaincy Service, for standing by our side as the ban was lifted, and also Commander Graham Beard RN and Commander Tim Kingsbury RN, passionate early advocates of LGBTQ equality.

Mark Eynon for his enthusiasm and support with the development of the book.

Dr Emma Vickers, of Liverpool John Moores University and Midshipman Adam Mason RNR, for their editorial support.

Jonathan Wright and Heather Williams at Pen and Sword Books, for being as passionate about this book as the authors from the day they saw the proposal, and every day since. Their hard work and enthusiasm got the writing team out of the trenches and over the line.

Linne Matthews, our copy editor, for her patience and persistence in support of the authors. She made these soldiers, sailors and air folks seem more competent as wordsmiths than might otherwise have been the case!

… and not least to all those partners, family, friends, allies and advocates who embraced, supported, inspired and championed our cause while standing by our sides. We will forever be grateful for the chance to be true, to be equal, to love and to serve.

Extracts from *This Queer Angel* by Elaine Chambers reproduced by kind permission of Unbound Digital.

All author royalties from the sale of this book will be donated to military and LGBT+ charities.

Foreword

by Admiral Lord West GCB DSC PC

I am honoured to have been invited to write the foreword to this groundbreaking book.

It comprises ten individual chapters, each written by a serviceman or woman who generously shares their experiences of being LGBT+ in the Armed Forces through times of intolerance and discrimination, and the subsequent changing of attitudes and legislation that have led to acceptance and equality.

Without exception, the stories are frank and revealing, and there is a deep poignancy about the double life that these individuals, and many others like them, were forced to live because of the rules and fear of discovery. There is now a new generation of LGBT+ serving men and women who know nothing of the old prejudices; their stories will be different, and my dearest wish is that they should be defined by their military service and not their gender, ethnicity or sexual orientation.

The world is more chaotic today than at any time during my fifty-four years of service. The dangers to our global rules-based system, which has ensured peace, security and prosperity since the Second World War, are significant and growing. The need for capable and effective Armed Forces is now greater than ever.

I know from years in command that to have a first-rate team one must recognise and use the unique talents that every member of one's ship's company, squadron or unit bring to the party, valuing their differences and the comradeship that binds them together. Only in that way can we enhance operational effectiveness such that we make our Armed Forces the best in the world.

History shows us that sexual orientation has no bearing on the performance of a warrior in battle; a case in point is Sir Michael Howard, a winner of the Military Cross, whose 1995 memorandum advocating change is reproduced in this book.

Let us be quite clear: over the years, indeed centuries, LGBT+ personnel have served with loyalty and distinction at every level in our Armed Forces. And yet for most of that time we did not accept the fact; we put our heads in the sand and pretended the situation did not exist.

In hindsight, it is shameful to accept that *gays* and *lesbians* were very publicly hounded and forced to end their service careers. Many were outed to their units, families and friends. In some cases, they were arrested and subjected to degrading medical examinations – leading to dismissal. When I became Naval Secretary in 1994, I was so disturbed by the treatment of individuals on the basis of an anonymous phone call that I put a stop to the SIB conducting such investigations.

Like the paradox of Heller's *Catch 22*, LGBT+ Forces personnel were classed as a threat to security because of the risk of blackmail by hostile intelligence services. Why were they at risk of blackmail? Because our system said it was wrong to be *gay*.

When in action, the last thing that entered my consciousness was the sexual orientation of any of my people. All I wanted to know was that they were giving of their utmost as part of my team to fight and win. I only discovered later that one of my best senior rates during our fighting in the Falklands was homosexual.

I am often told that LGBT+ personnel will be focused on being part of a 'homosexual community' rather than on their mates in the Forces, but I don't believe so. They belong with equal measure within the community with which they have trained and serve, whether in a ship or submarine, air squadron, or commando or army unit.

Whilst we can understand the reasons why the Armed Forces lagged behind in terms of social change, the acceptance of LGBT+ personnel took far too long and the harsh treatment that many endured is utterly regrettable.

I am delighted with the impartiality and objectivity that proliferates today. Forgetting the benefits for military capability, it was quite simply the right thing to do.

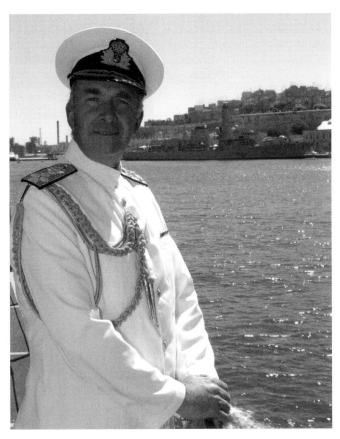

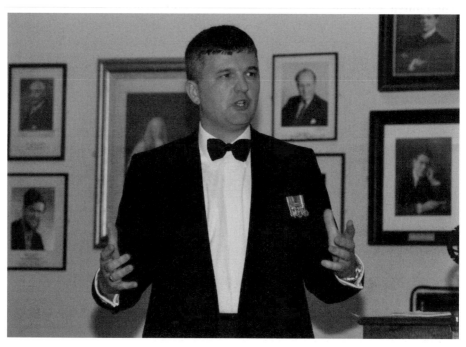

Craig Jones, at the Cambridge Union, March 2011.

Introduction

by Lieutenant Commander Craig Jones MBE Royal Navy

The United Kingdom, its people and its government, are universally proud of LGBTQ members of our Armed Forces who serve today with distinction at the front line of operations. These men and women are welcomed in their ships, squadrons and regiments, valued for their unique contribution, and their careers thrive. They fly fighter jets, command warships and submarines and they lead infantry units. They serve wherever our uniform is seen, their voices heard not with a whimper, but with a roar. They are defined by their military service, not their sexuality or gender identity, and they are part of a team that is respected throughout the world. Today's LGBTQ servicemen and women are protected by an inclusive Armed Forces Covenant, which offers a promise from our nation that those who stand in our protection in our hour of need, and their families, shall not go unnoticed in *their* hour of need. Our nation promises that they need not ask, we will be there for them. These are the stories of the LGBTQ warriors who are defined by their selflessness, dedication, hard work and courage. It is hard to remember a time when we were not rightly proud of them, but there was a time.

Today, those in the Armed Forces LGBTQ community live in an honourable peace from a dishonourable war. The 'gay ban' was an extraordinary breach of the Armed Forces Covenant by service chiefs, the impact of which was felt by thousands of our dearest and best. Perhaps most difficult to understand is how contrary the ban was to the peace, respect and freedoms our Armed Forces uphold.

Victory in this struggle was won by tall poppies trained in battle for a different fight, but who readily grabbed the baton and fought for the privilege of service. One of the greatest acts of courage is to say no, when all those about you say 'yes'. These men and women said 'no', and kept saying it until dissent was no more. As they were dismissed or as the first among equals, they walked into messes and wardrooms, briefing rooms and canteens with heads held high amidst a wider Armed Forces that was at first bewildered by the change. Today, perhaps we better understand the remarkable courage in their dignity.

To a great many people, the fact that the Armed Forces had a forty-five-year war with their gay community might today pass unnoticed. Social change has leapt forward at a pace that leaves the past in a fog, the origin and journey lost in the warmth of today's welcome. There is some reassurance in the surprise of many people at the fact that there really was a gay ban, so blistering has been the pace of change. These chapters record a history that is so at odds with where we find ourselves today that it is at times difficult to fathom. What is most striking about the Armed Forces' volte-face on LGBTQ equality is the distance travelled in so little time. In the mid-1990s, senior officers were placing open letters in national newspapers proclaiming the unacceptable damage that 'out' LGBTQ servicemen and women would have on operational effectiveness in military units. Today, those LGBTQ men and women help make us not the largest Armed Force in the world, but perhaps the best.

These chapters record the accounts of men and women who have served in every conflict including and since the Second World War, with careers and loves in constant discord. Some of these accounts are of beloved careers thrown on the fires, lost to our Armed Forces at the stroke of a pen: 'Services No longer Required'. Their story of the legal battles is a David and Goliath tale, with grit and determination that makes the protagonists of change worthy of a plinth in Parliament Square. In a case that is considered the most important human rights case of the twentieth century, they fought the United Kingdom government in every court in the land, winning victory in the European Court of Human Rights in the summer of 1999. They fought not for compensation, but for principle and for equality for those serving in the shadows, and for future generations. Winning this case was the first brick to fall in the wall of LGBTQ legislative inequality, trailblazing for the repeal of Section 28 and the Equal Treatment Directives of the Goods and Services Act.

Others of these stories are of the first amongst equals. Gay personnel who came out and stood tall in an ill-prepared Armed Forces, less than a handful of months after the government walked shamefaced from the European Court of Human Rights. LGBTQ servicemen and women in our Armed Forces quietly cheered as the ban was lifted, and then wept … and then got on with the job. The service of these resilient and often decorated and honoured lesbian, gay and transgender officers puts the ban in a harsh light.

Despite our best endeavours, however, and having cast the net far and wide for Bi voices, we are aware that this book records an LGbT history and not an LGBT+ history, and important voices remain unheard. The changes we and others have brought about have opened pathways for the full spectrum of love that exists in our communities, but we realise there is still a fight to be won. We stand at the side of the whole community, until one day everybody can truly be themselves.

In my service and in my life beyond the military, I have been privileged to meet some remarkable servicemen and women who embody all that is good about our Armed Forces. Their losses and the rigours they have faced will leave you dewy-eyed, their courage and triumphs will make your heart leap. Most importantly, their stories are a celebration of men and women with loyalty and love for our Armed Forces that have stood the test.

Chapter 1

Action Stations
Sub Lieutenant Edmund Hall
Royal Navy

It's not always possible to work out exactly when and where a political campaign began, but it couldn't really be easier to date the crusade to end the ban on gays serving in the military, and how perfectly romantic it is for the history books, because it started very appropriately at Pride in London in the summer of 1993.

It was a glorious and sunny Pride day that year, and I think it was my third Pride since I'd been sacked as a young officer from the Royal Navy for being gay. Rank Outsiders was the recently formed support group for lesbians and gay men set up to help when they got into trouble in the forces, and it had become a very important social group for those of us who had been dropped unceremoniously back into society with a badly tarnished CV. Rank Outsiders had a banner, and that became a focal point for lesbians and gay men with a military background attending Pride. Of course, back then, nobody wore their uniforms – serving people risked immediate arrest – and the

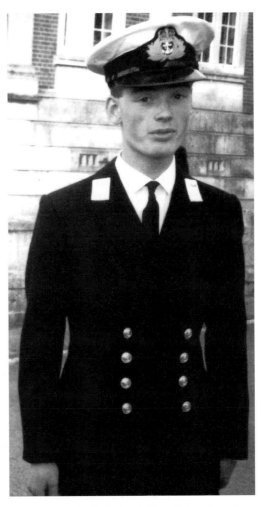

Midshipman Ed Hall, Royal Navy, full of hope for a naval career, which sadly wasn't to be.

police had on more than one occasion stopped marchers wearing some element of military dress and threatened them with arrest for impersonating a member of the Armed Forces. The rumour mill was rife with gossip that there was an ex-Army police officer in the Metropolitan Police who would arrest anyone he thought was wearing any military uniform.

I still had my blue-badged Navy beret then, now long since lost, and I wore that with a trendy T-shirt and shorts: it was what we would now call, with raised eyebrow, 'a bold look'. I glanced nervously at police officers as we passed them, but nobody approached me. We marched as a small group, and occasionally another marcher or spectator would stroll alongside us and nervously introduce themselves as a serving or retired member of the forces. They were scared, they were often lonely, and they wanted to know how to get in touch with the group. This was before the web, and before the MoD agreed to let anyone know that Rank Outsiders even existed. We had a helpline that we took turns to answer, and terrified members of the forces facing a police investigation or arrest would call us

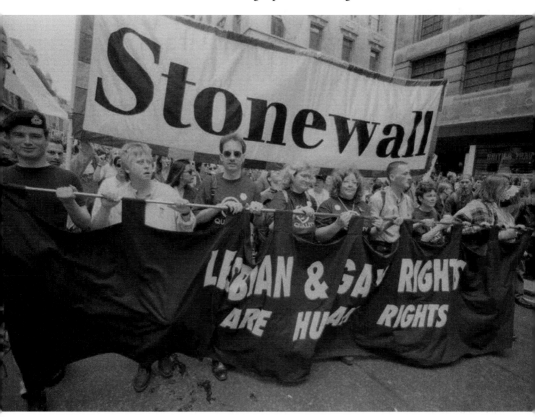

'Manning the barricades' at Pride and somewhat bravely wearing my beret … but with an eye out for the Military Police!

during the two hours a week we were open and ask for help. Frequent discussions took place about whether or not the calls were being secretly monitored by service police officers.

Only the bold or the very desperate would come to meet us so publicly, and for serving members the prospect of being seen was so terrifying that they would often rush out, take a phone number and hurriedly disappear back into the crowd.

RAF Sergeant Simon Ingram was one of those serving, and he was in the middle of a complex and ultimately terminal career crisis: suspended, under investigation and facing imminent dismissal. He marched with us, alongside his then partner, and I suspect he was probably the first serving member of the forces to march openly at Pride. I spoke to him that day and began a strong friendship that still continues.

I was in the very early days of my media career in 1993, and I was working as a freelance contributor for *The Independent*. The opportunity to write a story about Simon leapt out at me, but I was nervous about it, partly because of the risk for him, but also because my own career at that stage had steered well clear of gay stories that struck close to home. It was being gay that had seen me investigated and questioned by the Special Investigation Branch in 1988 and 1989, and the pain that had caused me and my family was very acute. It took a story as strong as Simon's to help me find my voice again, and he readily agreed to be interviewed. I believe it was the first newspaper story that had an interview with an open and named gay member of the Armed Forces, and it caught the imagination of the press and broadcasters. It quickly became obvious to me that there was real interest in the subject.

When Bill Clinton became US president in January 1993, he had done so on a promise to lesbians and gay men in the US Armed Forces that he would lift the ban on them serving, but after he won the election in November 1992, the phones began to ring, and the lobbying against his promise began. At its peak, the campaign to *prevent* the lifting of the ban generated a reported 68,000 phone calls to the White House and Pentagon in one day. The Clinton White House was not ready for this kind of campaign, and in the wake of the first Gulf War, was in no position to try to wrestle the Pentagon to the ground over it. The promise withered, and an irrational and poorly drafted replacement emerged – what would come to be known as 'Don't Ask, Don't Tell'. For the several prominent lesbians and gay men who had bravely come out after the Clinton victory, this was a disaster: they lost their jobs. In the first half of 1993, Bill Clinton's battles over his 'gays in the military' policy were front-page news across the world.

The impact of this unexpected development was also felt in the UK, and it was clear that the huge public controversy over the new American policy was driving media interest in what was happening in the British Armed Forces. I found an agent who was interested in representing me in writing a book on the subject: by the end of 1993, Random House had commissioned me and paid what seemed to me then like a huge advance. It was apparent that whatever reservations I may have had about becoming a reporter on gay issues, they were going to have to be set aside. I headed off to Australia, the Netherlands, and, of course, the United States to investigate. It was an amazing trip. I met extraordinary people and they often led me on to meet another and another: it was real-time journalism of the most exciting kind. I found myself with access to gay men and women serving at all levels of the forces, in occupations from the mundane to the secret and improbable. I finally found the proof, which I knew in my heart to be true, that lesbians and gay men were fighting in tanks, flying fighter aircraft, working in the intelligence agencies, guarding missile silos, in command of warships, managing personnel departments, maintaining aircraft, cooking, and working as doctors, nurses and dentists. It was clear that the presence of lesbians and gays, far from being what the MoD described as 'detrimental to good order and discipline', was in fact an integral (if often secret) part of the armed forces of all our allies.

Gay stories were at this stage becoming mainstream bread and butter for daytime television shows, news programmes, radio and newspapers. *Kilroy*, which was a daily *Jerry Springer*-like show, covered every story with a gay angle, and they often did so very well. During 1994, the lobbying group Stonewall began a major campaign to equalise the age of consent for gay sex, which was then set by law at a hugely discriminatory 21 years of age. I helped on that campaign as I was working in Parliament a great deal, and I began a ten-year relationship with Stonewall. The primary, almost sole focus of Stonewall, which was then just a small group of people in offices in Victoria's Greycoat Place, was the age of consent; the Armed Forces weren't even vaguely a Stonewall story or campaign priority.

For the support group Rank Outsiders, the rights and wrongs of political campaigning were a matter of considerable debate. The only work that Stonewall had done on the Armed Forces issue by 1994 was to help the founders of Rank Outsiders address an Armed Forces Select Committee meeting in the House of Commons some years earlier. I had by then joined the Rank Outsiders' committee and I wanted to make the lifting of the ban a major part of the group's aims, but whilst everyone was obviously sympathetic to the idea, there was a competing concern. Would the beginning of progress that was being made in 1) persuading the MoD to offer welfare support to those it was sacking, and 2) persuading the MoD to promulgate the contact details for Rank Outsiders be put at risk if they became openly political? The issue was debated amongst us at a meeting and forceful arguments against campaigning were put forward to a vote. To my surprise and some consternation, my proposal for Rank Outsiders to campaign for the ban to be lifted was voted down and the role of the organisation as a support and welfare group made clear.

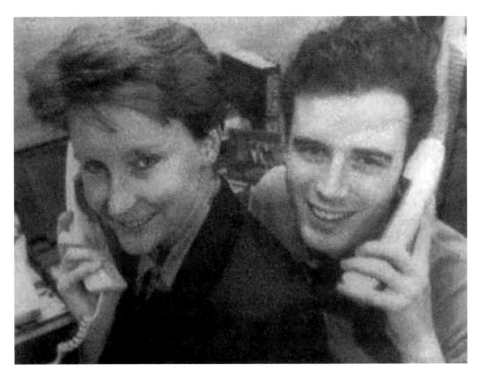

Me with Elaine Chambers, ready to answer the Rank Outsiders helpline, which was a lifeline for so many.

As a consequence of the vote against supporting a legal and political campaign, a sensible compromise was decided upon. Rank Outsiders agreed to support me in forming a new but separate body, the Armed Forces Legal Challenge Group, as a distinct but unrelated political group, and on a fresh piece of paper with a childishly large font on an Amstrad word processor, that's exactly what I did.

I finished the book in 1994, writing the last chapters in friends' spare bedrooms across the country as I had massively overspent the advance, which now didn't seem so big. In August 1994, I received a telephone call from *The Guardian* asking me about the cases in the book, what was happening in the UK, and whether Don't Ask, Don't Tell was the next step likely to be implemented here. I answered the questions with the Home Editor at some length, but the next day, to my huge surprise, I found that the front-page headline story was about gays in the military, and when I read the bold lines at the bottom of the article, 'A Naval Officer's Story, Page 3', I wondered who it was. I turned the page and found out. It was me.

It was August, so of course real stories were thin on the ground, but the charged atmosphere of the Clinton failure to lift the US ban made this immediately a much bigger story than I realised. The story in *The Guardian* predicted that the

US drama was about to start here, not least as I had said a legal challenge was likely. The phone went mad. The story was covered on the BBC's *One O'Clock News*, Radio 4's *World at One* and *PM*, Radio 1's *Newsbeat*, *ITV News* and *Channel 4 News*, and newspaper reporters from the USA, Tokyo and Sydney wanted to interview me. I couldn't cope and asked Simon Ingram to join me in Manchester to help do all these interviews. A news agency photograph of us walking along a Manchester canal went around the world, and by late afternoon, as we finished talking to the *Chicago Sun-Times*, the BBC was asking if I could appear that evening on *Newsnight* in London. They flew me down, gave me a suit to wear, and I found myself debating the ban on gays serving in the military with John Wilkinson MP, Chairman of the Armed Forces Defence Select Committee. Just a day earlier, I had been sitting in a borrowed kitchen writing the last chapters of the book, and putting together letters that sacked servicemen and women could pass to their lawyers explaining the campaign. Now I was in BBC Television Centre arguing about the ban with people who actually had the power to change it.

In twenty-four hours we had gone from a germ of an idea for a British campaign to lift the ban on lesbians and gays serving in the military, to a new reality that the campaign did exist and was being listened to ... and it had happened, quite literally, overnight. Shortly after midnight I checked into the Hilton hotel by the Holland Park roundabout in London, at the BBC's cost, and sat down to think through the madness of the day. I phoned my mother, who had just heard me on BBC Radio 4's *Midnight News*, and she was very angry and upset at hearing what she saw as our private family issues aired so publicly. I was starting to become aware how selfish and single-minded a campaigner had to be, even when the personal cost was high.

The book, *We Can't Even March Straight*, was finished by the end of 1994, and by then I'd been in touch with dozens, if not hundreds of people who had been affected by the ban. I wanted to find the best cases, and the lawyers who would represent them. People wrote to me, they called me, they got in touch through solicitors and through Rank Outsiders; in the end, I think we had almost a hundred potential cases to bring.

This needed pro bono legal work, as we had little or no resources to make this happen. Despite the huge publicity we had now achieved, I hadn't actually raised any money whatsoever to bring a case. But by this stage I had joined the Stonewall management group and began to lobby for the case to be supported by Stonewall. There was real resistance to this at first, and as we went into 1995, I knew that I still had to persuade the gay establishment that this was a campaign worth supporting. I did that in the only way I really understood, by keeping the story on television, radio and in the newspapers. I knew that if this continued to be the biggest gay story on the news, then even the hard-left, anti-military lesbian and gay campaigning establishment would eventually have to support us, despite their proud Greenham Common and CND march histories.

The momentum began to build, and one article I wrote in March 1995 stands out to me, as it mentions two of the four people who went on to become the test cases. I rather like the headline, which I'm afraid was not mine but the work of a smart subeditor, 'Stop the Generals Invading the Bedroom'.

The book came out in May 1995, and I somehow persuaded the publishers to rent HMS *Belfast* for the book launch. We created a very public debate, hosted by *The Today Programme*'s Peter Hobday, in which Peter Tatchell opposed the idea that gays should serve in the military. The dispute on this issue with Peter was emblematic of the issue I had with many of the other members of the Stonewall management group. They saw *coming out* as itself a wider form of social *liberation*, in which, to them, service in the military struck a jarring and discordant note. I think this line of thought continues to this day in other political discussions, where there seems to be a belief that because you are gay, you ought therefore to be of a lightly socialist bent, and that coming out is itself a process that makes you more politically correct. How can gays vote for Trump? Or Brexit? Or the Conservative Party? This divide is much more than philosophical, as a few months after I published *We Can't Even March Straight*, Peter Tatchell published his anti-military response, *We Don't Want to March Straight*.

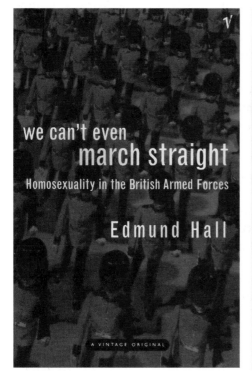
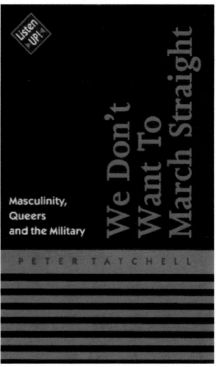

My book, *We Can't even March Straight*, and Peter Tatchell's rebuff – he later saw the light!

As the Armed Forces Legal Challenge Group moved in 1995 from my Amstrad word processor to the real world, we had to fight not only the traditional military establishment, but also the gay liberation movement establishment and its proud Clause 28 successors who found it almost impossible to reconcile their history of anti-establishment campaigning with support for men and women who had fought in the Gulf War, or served on nuclear submarines, or who proudly wore medals for their service in the Falklands. At times I felt I had become a sort of social translator, interpreting the language and culture of one group for the benefit and understanding of the other.

In the run-up to the book launch, I borrowed the Stonewall offices in Greycoat Place to hold a meeting for sacked service people, their lawyers and representatives. The meeting was promoted and supported by Rank Outsiders, who, despite their formal distancing from my campaign, had proved to be stout and determined supporters of it. I had worked closely with a London human rights firm in 1991 and 1992 on a case involving Channel 4 and a series of interviews they had conducted with an alleged terrorist, as my very first production company was by then advising Channel 4's programme *Dispatches* on the validity and truthfulness of the interviews. Bindmans was the firm representing the programme maker, and one of their lawyers, Stephen Grosz, had met me on several occasions.

We needed to find a law firm that would bundle up the cases and identify those that I could use to persuade Stonewall to back us: I was surprised and delighted when the relationships between the senior partners at Bindmans and Stonewall's leadership were made clear to me. I knew instantly that we had a law firm interested that had serious human rights credentials and the personal relationships that are often so important to achieving pro bono, deferred or 'no win, no fee' representation. Once the meeting had taken place, I also got to meet Maddy Rees of Tyndallwoods in Birmingham, who was also determined that her firm would support and represent cases. Between these two firms, and with these highly credible and passionate lawyers on board, we were able to invite potential claimants to contact them, and we finally had the concrete beginnings of a real legal fight.

We needed cases that involved both officers and other ranks, and, of course, both men and women, and they needed to be cases of clear-cut discrimination; we tried to avoid cases where discipline issues or complex personal problems had emerged. In reality it was a ruthless exercise in assessing both the cases and the individuals. Obviously we knew that the ban had itself been the cause of so many complex problems for people affected – something I knew all too well from my own experience – but in choosing the cases to take forward, we had to avoid problems of absence without leave, insubordination, sexual activity on a base or ship, successful blackmail or anything else that could distract from the simple message we wanted to carry to the courts. That truth was harsh. At times it felt as though I was judging the conduct of people who had found themselves in an impossible position and I recall a few challenging conversations with some whose cases weren't chosen. I was conscious of potential charges of hypocrisy, too, as for a while I had run away from dealing with my own situation just six years earlier.

These are the difficult moments in political campaigns that only years later you allow yourself to think about and meditate on the pain that the process caused, but at the time, as a campaigner, you simply plough ahead, maybe conscious of but strangely unaffected by the pain you have caused by telling someone else that their case isn't good enough, and knowing that's true about your own case too.

The year before, I had watched close up and from the inside how Stonewall's age of consent campaign had nearly torn apart the lives of the three young men who had risked prosecution to bring the absurdity of the 21-year-old age of consent to the public's attention, even to the extent of handing themselves in to the police for breaking the law. I knew from my own experience the previous August how dramatic the press attention could be when the spotlight found you, and I also knew how much that had upset my family. But if we were to win the battle, I knew it was only going to be partly in the courts. We had to win the battle for the public mood too, and I remember saying that we needed to look and sound like members of the Armed Forces in every interview and every photograph. It was why I had insisted on wearing a suit to appear on *Newsnight*, to the consternation of the researcher who had to find me one as I flew down to London at the BBC's expense. I was sure that by appearing to be the sort of men and women you envisage in the forces, we could persuade people to look again and think why on earth would you sack somebody like that? The lead cases needed to be strong people, with simple cases, ready to face the intense flash of cameras and cope with the scrutiny into their private lives that would inevitably follow.

The next four years would prove to be very tough for the men and women who became our cases. They were very different people, some of whom took to the media spotlight and enjoyed it, and some of whom hated it. Deep and prolonged critical attention was going to stay with them throughout, and at the same time, they were all dealing with dramatic changes and often periods of personal crisis in their private lives. After all, they weren't just gay superheroes and role models; they had to cope with being sacked from a career that for all of them was their hard-won dream.

By the early spring of 1995, Stonewall was on board and ready to fund a judicial review, the four clear lead cases had been agreed, and the solicitors prepared to bundle and support the other cases pro bono or on a 'no win, no fee' basis were in place. We had an initial list of about sixty also ready to sue. Finally, in the spring of 1995, we got ready for court.

David Pannick QC, now Lord Pannick of Article 50 legal challenge fame, was to lead the case. He says he never had any doubt about the merits of the case, but

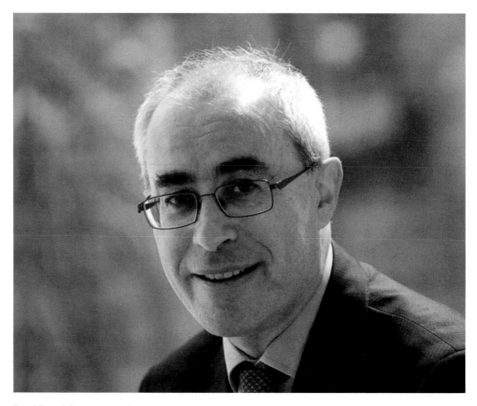

Lord Pannick – we were lucky to have in our corner the best legal advocate of his generation.

had serious reservations about whether it could be resolved in the British courts. The case was a judicial review of the decisions the MoD policy had led to, which was the dismissal of these four members of the Armed Forces for no other reason than their sexual orientation: Duncan Lustig-Prean had been a high-flying young Royal Navy lieutenant commander, reportedly destined for a distinguished career; Jeanette Smith was a hard-working RAF nurse who wanted no limelight and felt increasingly uncomfortable in the public eye; Graeme Grady had held extremely sensitive positions in the RAF, including spells working in intelligence roles at the British Embassy in Washington, and was a shy but determined man with the support of his ex-wife and children; and Royal Navy sailor John Beckett, who really only ever wanted someone to give him back the job he didn't understand why he'd lost. They were very different, with diverse family circumstances, and lived in different parts of the UK. Some needed financial assistance even to be able to attend court.

Of the four cases, Duncan and Graeme had been part of the earliest discussions about legal action, and Birmingham solicitor Maddy Rees had come to the Armed Forces Legal Challenge Group through her support for Jeanette in September

1994. Their stories were already in my book and I felt that we knew them and their experiences so well that we could campaign and confidently tell them again and again. John was the only one of the four who came to us new, and it took time for the others to bring him into the team. As the case went on it was John and Jeanette who were most uncomfortable with the limelight, and it took a few arguments with Stonewall to ensure that funding was available to help get them to court, find somewhere for them to stay, and make sure they were looked after. It has struck me ever since that political campaign groups can easily lose the human touch, and when I look online, I can barely find the names of those who put their lives on the line for the various campaigns of the 1990s. I feel rather ashamed of that.

History now is told through the web, and our 'gays in the military' campaign predates that. There are versions of the history of the epochal gay political campaigns of the 1990s littered around the online world that make amusing or depressing reading to those of us who were there, and that is as true of the age of consent campaign as it is of this one. As a community we haven't learned to thank and remember those who fought for our rights, and whose sacrifice was given in public and often at great personal cost. Not one of the names of any of the individuals who brought these cases in the 1990s even results in a hit if you search for them on the Stonewall website today. Our collective history has been partially erased or lost, and when writing this I used both Google and the Stonewall website to try to find out which year it was that we won the Stonewall Award for our campaign. The award ceremony took place in the Royal Albert Hall in the late 1990s. Elton John, Boy George, Ian McKellen and other stars of stage and screen performed to a full house. We assembled with the Police Association to collect our awards, and as we walked down the aisles to the stage, the whole auditorium stood and cheered us to the rafters. But now, none of the winners or any of the awards from that crucial decade are listed anywhere. It's almost as though it never happened.

But at the time, if we wanted to win the wider battle of hearts and minds, we had to show who we were; we had to show the public that the decision to sack us was wrong and that the four subjects of the lead case were exactly the sort of men and women everyone would want to see serving their country. The very first time they were introduced to the press we needed to have photographs ready, so we got them together at the main doors of the MoD. It was an example of the careful plans we had to make, and how much detail was needed to make sure events like this could happen. I tried to ensure that the 'Gays-in-the-Military Four' would feel supported and ready. Jeanette was terrified and needed the support of her girlfriend to cope with the stresses of the day after travelling down from Scotland, whereas Duncan turned up in his full dress naval uniform with aiguillettes (the extravagant gold braid worn by staff officers to very senior officers) on his left shoulder, and a sword. He proceeded to walk in and out of the entrance to Horse

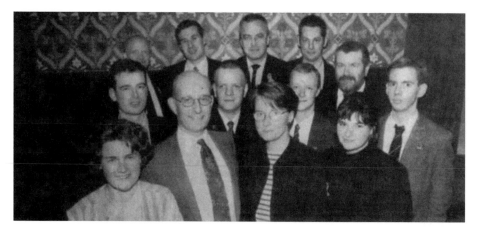

Me with Elaine Chambers, Patrick Lyster-Todd and many others at Westminster, firing shots across the bow of Parliament.

Guards, which meant that the famous guards on horseback were required to salute: we thought that funny at the time. As the day and the press conferences ended, I realised how tough the blending of these very different people, and the needs that they had, was going to be. Trying to support them and keep them together was going to be a major part of the next few months and years.

Lord Pannick recalls that from the very beginning of proceedings he felt that the merits of the other side were very weak, but they were cases that would be difficult to win in the UK courts. Even twenty years later, when he talks about the case you can tell how strongly he felt that there was a moral as well as legal issue in his mind when he took them to the High Court. I remember that very first hearing in May 1995. I was sitting a few rows behind the barristers and remember being fascinated by Lord Pannick's extraordinary recall of the right document and his ability to turn to the correct reference as the formidable legal banter with the judges followed. I could immediately see that this type of litigation was, in part, an intellectual sport, however serious the subject, but that we also had a real superstar at work.

The key obstacle to winning the case at that stage, however, wasn't the moral argument, and to a significant extent it wasn't really a black-and-white legal one either. The case hinged on a so-called legal test in public law known as the Wednesbury principle. This little-known but vital legal precedent was at the heart of the case as it made its way to Europe. The principle it refers to is one that states a decision made by a public servant cannot be found to be irrational unless the decision is so irrational as to be considered *perverse in all the circumstances*. As Lord Pannick explained to us then, and again when he recalled the case with me twenty years later, this is an incredibly high test to reach in a court. To pass the test and convince a court that the government is wrong, you have to persuade

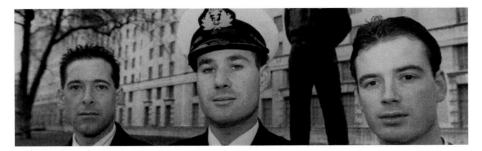

Me with Graeme Grady and Duncan Lustig-Prean, very definitely 'outside' the Ministry of Defence.

a judge that no rational person could come to the view that the government has come to, in any circumstances. In colloquial terms, you have to show that the decision is *bonkers*, not just wrong.

When the first stage of the case was lost, the judge's reasoning was significant, and it supported all that David Pannick and the solicitors had said. In his judgment, Lord Justice Simon Brown strongly rejected the MoD's arguments for maintaining the ban, but he said that the court could not overturn a policy that had been approved by Parliament, even though he recognised the ban involved a fundamental breach of human rights. The Wednesbury principle had not been met.

Lord Justice Brown went on in what Stonewall's chief executive Angela Mason described at the time as 'extraordinary lengths for a judge' to give his personal opinion on the ban: 'The tide of history is against the Ministry. Prejudices are breaking down ... It seems to me improbable, whatever this court may say, that the existing policy can survive much longer.'

And so, as the case went on and the public debates heated up, that was the legal ground where the government sought to defend itself, by demonstrating to the court and the country that the policy of sacking lesbians and gay men was rational and based on evidence. It was that requirement that caused the MoD to launch the next salvo in its attempt to justify and keep the ban, which was the announcement of an unexpected 'thorough internal review' of the 'gays in the military' policy by the MoD.

The years 1995 and 1996 were set to be a period during which the 'gays in the military' story never really left the news, because just as the case was rejected by the first court and work began on the appeal, the House of Commons started holding select committee meetings into the ban as part of their five-yearly examination of the Armed Forces Discipline Acts. In response to the need for new evidence for the court, and for the questioning they were shortly to face from MPs, the MoD created a task force called the Homosexuality Policy Assessment Team (HPAT), which was asked to examine the policy and make recommendations about its future.

The HPAT report turned out to be a last-gasp attempt by the old guard to prevent the ban being lifted, the content of which would have been funny had it not been so serious. The research consisted of a series of focus groups and questionnaires, and the whole process was managed through the chain of command, ensuring from the outset that it would have been a brave service member who would have spoken out against the official policy. It was clear from the outset that the HPAT team was set up for the primary purpose of creating evidence to support the ban, but even the most cynical observers were left a little surprised by the bizarre end product.

In examining the policy, the HPAT team approach was to identify all the potential issues that the presence of lesbians and gay men could cause. The report acknowledged at the start that gay people could and had served with distinction, but the HPAT research works clearly towards a single conclusion, which is that the ability of the Armed Forces to be an effective *fighting force* would be diminished by the presence of homosexuals. There was an immediate problem with that approach, which was that some people are in reality less gay than others, or at least they are in the sense of not being out. If gay people could serve effectively in secret, that would be an irrational conclusion to reach in support of a wholesale ban, and so the HPAT team identified nine different types of homosexual that required researching. These types of homosexuals varied largely on the basis of how out or how closeted they were. It led some of us to note that, according to the MoD, there were more types of homosexual than there were colours on the rainbow flag.

The full list of types of homosexual who pose a risk to the effectiveness of a fighting force that the MoD examined was: homosexual activist, flamboyant homosexual, declared homosexual, open homosexual, strongly suspected homosexual, suspected homosexual, covert homosexual, known homosexual, and a non-practising or celibate homosexual. It was never clear quite how or why these distinctions were helpful, but this approach successfully added a gloss of academic rigour and complexity to an already bizarre piece of research.

The report was made up of analysis from questionnaires and a small number of focus group meetings held in semi-formal sessions of half a dozen service people in a room where they were asked what they thought or felt about the potential presence of homosexuals in the Armed Forces. They were asked *by* the Armed Forces what they thought about the policy *of* the Armed Forces, and all were given the contact details of a professional psychologist in case they needed to discuss the traumatic impact of being in the focus group session or filling in the written questionnaire. At that stage, in 1995, the respondents to a MoD questionnaire about homosexuality were being offered more emotional support and care than those who were being sacked.

The legitimacy of the approach and validity of the data gathered was questioned harshly by MPs, and ultimately, the European Court of Human Rights would clearly identify all the flaws and weaknesses in the HPAT report. But it was enough to convince the British courts that the ban was not *perverse in all the circumstances*, and so the case was doomed to fail in the face of these early hurdles. The Minister of State for the Armed Forces Nicholas Soames eventually placed copies of the HPAT report in the House of Commons library, and he told the House of Commons: 'The team's assessment is that any relaxation of the existing policy is likely to have a detrimental effect on operational effectiveness. For that reason, the government will continue to support the existing policy of excluding homosexuals from the Armed Forces.'

The detrimental effects that the minister was worried about were pretty shocking, and the report gave space to quotes from the service people they had surveyed. It's important to remember that the MoD was using this 'evidence' to support their policy: in other words, the actions and threats contained in the quotes were used to underpin government policy. The quotes include: 'Homosexuals would get beaten up – I'd smash their face in.'

The report wants to make sure that the reader is left in no doubt how serious this threat would be, and it lists the unique types of violence associated with each branch of the military. In the Army, the report explains, the preferred method of assault is termed 'bed-ending', which consists of striking sleepers with hard objects wrapped in towels. Gay Navy personnel can look forward to blows with Samson bars (metal bars clipped next to each hatch) when moving around ship, and we learn that in the Royal Air Force, the tradition is 'taking someone behind the hangar', which at least has the benefit of potential as a *double entendre*.

So as 1995 wore on, we had a campaign fighting on three fronts: firstly, to win the court case; secondly, to win political support for the lifting of the ban in the Armed Forces Select Committee; and finally, to win over hearts and minds in the court of popular opinion. The Gays-in-the-Military Four began to develop their public identities and, increasingly, they became the voices of the campaign. Those committee members of Rank Outsiders who had worried about the reputation of the organisation two years earlier were now front and centre of the media campaigns, and several gave evidence to the select committee. The fears about the damage such campaigning would do were now less of a concern, and the campaigning became mainstream. Duncan Lustig-Prean became the organisation's first head of campaigns.

We had now become part of the political and media establishment, our phone numbers were on newspaper and television correspondents' speed dial, and we all worked to keep the story alive. I wrote columns or op-ed pieces constantly, and I became a pre-planned staple commentator of the local phone-in radio show.

On one memorable night I completely forgot that I was on a phone-in show on BBC radio across the north of England after the 10.00 pm news. I remembered at 9.45 pm while sitting in Wagamama's noodle restaurant in Soho. After sprinting to Broadcasting House, it became clear I did not have enough time to get to the studio and so I dialled in from the security desk in reception, sitting cross-legged on the floor behind the guards. That was the only time I got to debate the ban with a defence minister on air: the appearances were so frequent and routine that I had actually nearly forgotten about one.

We also spent a lot of time at Westminster lobbying MPs and members of the House of Lords. We had become the RAC or British Heart Foundation of gay campaigns, a well-known, respected and legitimate voice, largely made up of people who looked and spoke like *normal* people. It was a controversial time to do that, as HIV activism was also at its height, and as Terrence Higgins Trust became the RAC of gay health concerns, Peter Tatchell's activist group OutRage! was taking *queer* protest to the streets. I joined Peter and his group on a few of their breathtaking actions, for example, storming a church in Victoria that was hosting a rock concert for a gay conversion ministry, and I also reported on the occasion when he rented a pink armoured personnel carrier to drive around Trafalgar Square during a rally for Hizb ut-Tahrir, the gay-hating Islamist group led by Omar Bakri Mohammed. Alongside those extraordinary, creative, genius protests, our own pinstriped lobbying seemed rather tame, strangely subversive and counter-culture, and there were people who wanted to take protests to military and naval bases and to aim stunts at the MoD itself. I spent several long nights in 1996 and 1997 trying to convince fellow campaigners of my view that this battle would be won quickest by presenting a face that the Armed Forces would want to recognise and serve with, and we largely succeeded. There never was a pink tank covered with sacked gay soldiers on top driving around Aldershot playing Gloria Gaynor and dancing in their underwear – although the idea was seriously considered.

My role as translator between these types of campaigning had its sharpest moment when Stonewall chose to launch a major fundraising campaign based on our case. Nothing wrong with that, you might think, but they did so in a way that meant I had to intervene. Without discussion or consultation with us, Stonewall had commissioned a photo shoot of sexy guys in military uniforms wrapped in rainbow flags and showing some chiselled torso. They had printed thousands of postcards with these images, and they were being distributed nationally to elicit donations. The models in the photographs were wearing mixed foreign and weird rented uniforms from a fancy-dress shop, with US Navy caps, and the very handsome pouting figures (whilst obviously very inviting) represented exactly the image I had been trying so hard to avoid. I knew that if these postcards were distributed amongst those whose anti-gay voices were so clear in the HPAT report, they would only go to prove the horrifying image in those homophobes' minds of the reality they imagined of gay service people.

This was probably the only time in the whole campaign I really lost my temper. As I look back, it reminds me how isolated and tiny our campaign was, as Stonewall had felt able to create a huge national fundraising exercise and commission a studio photo shoot with models dressed as soldiers and sailors without it even occurring to them to discuss it with us. Nearly a quarter of a century later, Stonewall caused similar upset with the organisers of Pride events up and down the country when they closed a national sponsorship deal with Primark to sell Pride-labelled merchandise, without making any attempt to discuss it with any Pride organisers first or offer to share the money. The harsh reality is that arrogance is part of the armoury that campaigners use; it is part of the confidence of being right that you need to keep going and it was something I had been deeply alert to when we chose the examples to take forward with the case. Maybe it remains an issue for Stonewall, a very important body for the gay community, but one that whilst seeking to *represent*, perhaps sometimes fails to *listen*.

The multi-pronged approach meant that the political work continued too, and several of us gave evidence to the Armed Forces Select Committee. We had strong support from individuals in both main parties, but inevitably, much more resistance to change from the Conservatives. Labour's shadow defence secretary had said to me clearly and repeatedly that he supported a lifting of the ban, and the select committee asked some very searching questions of the MoD. For a moment in 1995 and 1996, it felt as though we were on the cusp of change: as though the case might win, that Parliament might change the law, or that a change of government would mean a change in policy.

Sadly, that moment of optimism was short-lived, and we again found ourselves on the back foot after the first and second stages of the judicial review in the courts failed; the MoD produced the absurd HPAT report, and the select committee accepted that evidence. The ban was still in place, people were still losing their jobs, and investigations by the service police forces were still ongoing. But despite those negatives, some things had already begun to change. During the period of the campaign the MoD had agreed that people who were sacked would no longer lose their pensions, they had agreed to share the helpline number for Rank Outsiders with people being dismissed, and Armed Forces charities like SSAFA were beginning to take the issue seriously. The bright media spotlight had made the battle over the ban much more public and tense, but in some significant ways, it also had a humanising affect on the still discriminatory process. People were much less likely to be searched, or to be kept in confinement, or be persuaded to attend interviews with representation that was far from independent. The ban was still in place, but even its strongest supporters now spoke of the evidence of service by lesbians and gays with some respect. The law itself may still have been in place, but its reasoning – its very *raison d'être* – was coming apart. As the 1997 General Election came, and the Labour Party, with its clearly stated promise to us to lift the ban, was on the home straight, most of us thought the final battle in the campaign was now just months away.

By this stage I had been campaigning for nearly five years. I'd written the book and appeared on every radio and television show possible, most of them on multiple occasions. I'd taken late-night cars or trains to and from Birmingham, Manchester, Cardiff, Bristol, Norwich, Glasgow, Leeds and Newcastle to debate the issue on television. I'd been a speaker at both the Oxford and Cambridge unions. I had spoken at universities across the country, from Southampton to Nottingham. I had become the gay military expert on BBC Radio and a regular reporter on BBC Radio 5 Live's groundbreaking and award-winning programme *Out This Week*. I was the gay military feature writer in *The Independent* and a regular feature writer in most other papers too. I had argued with both Rank Outsiders and Stonewall to make the campaign happen in the first place, and I'd worked to keep the whole thing on track. I think the instant and powerful rejection of the promises Labour politicians had made to us when they came to power was the moment I felt I'd come to the end of the road. It was now clear that the only way the ban would be lifted was through the court case itself, and that was in the hands of excellent lawyers, supported by Stonewall, and one or two of the people that the case was centred on had themselves become very good media campaigners, Duncan in particular.

For the first time, I became more of a spectator, and for the last eighteen months I watched with pride but from a distance as the case finally made it to Strasbourg. My biggest regret is that I didn't go to see the case and judgments in the European Court of Human Rights, but I heard amazing stories of the excitement of it all. David Pannick told me that there was one obviously hostile judge on the panel, and he directed much of his thirty minutes of time to Judge Loukis Loucaides from Cyprus. During the hearing the judge interrupted to ask David Pannick what would happen if his client was in the Army, on manoeuvres, up a mountain, and there was a sudden snowstorm. The legal teams looked puzzled, but the judge continued to explain that the soldiers would obviously have to huddle together for warmth, and how could that be possible with Mr Pannick's client?

David Pannick was pondering a response when he received a note passed forward from one of the legal team that read, 'Tell him that if it was that cold, none of them would want to get their knobs out!'

The eminent Mr Pannick chose not to relay that to the judge.

The judges spent the next few months considering their verdict, and finally, on 27 September 1999, the ruling was given: the ban was illegal; the government had failed to respect their rights to privacy and family life. For a government that had not proved brave enough to do it itself, this ruling provided the cover they needed to finally instruct the MoD to get on with it. The change came like an express train, just as we had all said it would, because if there's one group of people in Britain who are mostly likely to do what they are told, it's the Armed Forces. It was obvious that the MoD had prepared properly, and consulted in advance with others, but even so, the speed of change really was phenomenal.

I had already left the campaigning behind, and I watched with fascination from afar as an uneasy transfer of power took place. Shortly after the verdicts were announced, I was deeply honoured to be awarded Rank Outsiders' Peter Clarke Award for the creation and success of the Armed Forces Legal Challenge Group at a celebratory dinner in Bristol. But the future role of Rank Outsiders was becoming unclear. It was time for the voice of gay military life to move on from the voluntary, passionate and amateur Rank Outsiders to become a formal part of MoD life: people in uniforms whose job is to be pro-gay and supportive. I watched as some lesbians and gay men quietly went back to the jobs from which they had not long before been sacked. I felt some empathy with the obvious challenges the MoD and the voluntary gay groups had in communicating with each other; it was oddly reminiscent of the challenges I'd faced at the beginning as I tried to explain to Greenham Common veterans why this fight was important. One sacked naval serviceman even went back to a senior job on a nuclear submarine. I thought for a moment about my own career, and I even looked at some leaflets and websites and considered rejoining, before deciding that media was now my home. That passion

PETER CLARKE AWARD 1999

FOR OUTSTANDING SERVICE TO RANK OUTSIDERS

Edmund Hall

Since its inception, Rank Outsiders has had two main avenues of work, namely the provision of Welfare and Support services and the campaign to overturn the blanket ban against gay men, lesbians and bisexuals serving in the United Kingdom Armed Forces, the latter being pursued through both political pressure and legal challenge.

From the earliest days of his membership, Edmund Hall's interest in socio-political affairs has enabled him to work diligently on our behalf in a number of areas, but principally in the background of our campaign.

In recognition of his outstanding work, and in particular for his initiative in setting up the Armed Forces Legal Challenge Group, which bore such spectacular fruits at the European Court of Human Rights this year, Rank Outsiders is proud to honour Edmund Hall with the 1999 Peter Clarke Award.

....
Robert Ely, President

....
Steve Johnston, Chair

Recognition of my work with Rank Outsiders.

for the sea is still there, though, and my sixteen years of service as a volunteer crewmember in the RNLI and my hobby of racing yachts perhaps suggests there's still a bit of that young Royal Navy midshipman in me somewhere.

I can date the moment I realised what the change really meant as clearly as I can date the day it all started. It was at the Stonewall Awards in 2005, held at the Victoria and Albert Museum in London, and I had gone as a private guest with no visible or formal link to Stonewall or the campaign. The winner of Employer of the Year was the Royal Navy, the award collected on stage by the Second Sea Lord. I had no previous warning that the Navy was even shortlisted: I had really just gone, like most guests, for the free champagne. As I sat in the crowd and saw the announcement, I was sitting next to a group of people who knew me, but they had no idea about what I'd been up to ten years earlier, and they were deeply concerned when I burst into tears. All the emotions and passion and anger and pain from the days I had spent under arrest for being gay in 1988 at HMS Nelson in Portsmouth before I was sacked; all the times over five years I had tried to spin the homophobes' arguments back at them on radio and television programmes; all the late-night calls from terrified people we had handled on our helpline from phone boxes they had driven for miles to call us from – all of it came back to me visually and physically and left me short of breath. I think it was that night that I finally dealt in my heart with what had happened to me, and since then I've been able to look back on the campaign with pride, and without embarrassment at my own screwed-up career, and I have been able to look my military friends in the eye and say, yes, maybe I didn't have a long and distinguished naval career, but at least I did do something about it.

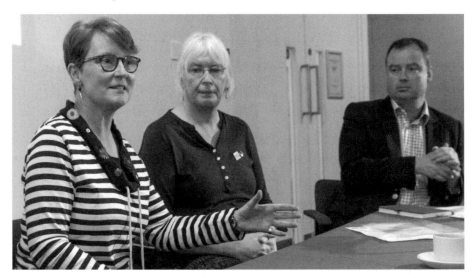

Me with Elaine Chambers (left) and Caroline Paige.

Chapter 2

Absent Friends
Lieutenant Commander Patrick Lyster-Todd
Royal Navy

This part of my life began back in 1970 while in my third year boarding at St Edward's School in Oxford – a first division English boys' public school (now co-ed), not quite up there with Eton and Harrow but in good company with the likes of Stowe and Radley, Wellington and Marlborough. While we didn't really turn out prime ministers, as Teddies' boys (as we were known) we had – and have – a reputation of being reliable and steady, occasionally a bit maverick; always someone good to have on one's side. This, sadly, was writ all too well on the wooden plaques that lined both sides of the chapel walls whose names picked out in gold mark that Teddies turned out a greater proportion of young men who answered the call of their country in the Great War than any other independent school in Britain and, in turn, who paid for that honour.

It didn't really stop there, either, and in some strange way the school also produced some of Britain's and the RAF's greatest aviators, from both world wars: Arthur Banks, Adrian Warburton, Geoffrey de Havilland, Louis Strange, Guy Gibson and Douglas Bader. While a leading seaman in the school's Combined Cadet Force in 1971, I was even inspected by that amazing

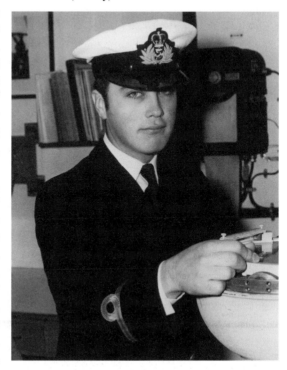

As a sub lieutenant at Britannia Royal Naval College, Dartmouth, 1975.

man himself, Group Captain Douglas Bader, whose gait (he had two false legs as, indeed, he had had during the Battle of France and, later, the Battle of Britain) was barely discernible. Glancing at my name tally, he had smiled and remarked, 'Got a bit of a list to starboard, have we?' – noticing my tendency to not quite square off my shoulders.

For some today, it is fair game to take a pop at Britain's 'private school elite' – privileged, possibly, but at times you'd think that we were a hotbed of upper-class twits, selfish by nature and gay by inclination. The truth, as ever, is far different, but the biggest difference was marked less by the facilities, the emphasis on sport (we had over a dozen playing fields, two sports centres and two pools) and us pupils but by the teaching excellence we were exposed to. This enabled academically mediocre individuals like me to achieve, often beyond our potential and, especially, to develop a mindset that was independent and self-reliant while also firmly committed to the benefits of teamwork. The key to superior teaching lay, of course, in the staff themselves: superbly skilled, often brilliant, sometimes slightly mad, eccentric and, occasionally, totally barking. They helped shape the person I am today, generally, I hope, for good.

One known to several generations of Teddies' boys was Joe McPartlin (or JJMcP). He was my O level geography master, but also a talented rugby coach, Combined Cadet Force commanding officer, wit, house tutor and raconteur par excellence. He was a complete one-off – not just inspirational on the rugby pitch ('I've seen better centres in a box of Milk Tray') but truly unique in the classroom. Each lesson was something to look forward to, and laughs, invariably involving some anecdote or escapade, often revolving around some misfortunate, were guaranteed. The stories – many, knowing Joe, not apocryphal – were legion and often passed down by parent alumni to sons as if a Patek timepiece. My favourite concerned his interview with the Warden (headmaster) when he'd first applied to join the Common Room. Joe was convinced that, following an indifferent performance, what tipped the balance into being offered a place was the tie he was wearing, with its initials of 'OUDS' (assumed, by the Warden, as standing for the Oxford University Dramatic Society), whereas what couldn't be seen, beneath the 'V' of his jersey, were the three crossed darts. In later years, returning to the school as an old boy, often when acting as a mentor to a sixth-former considering the Royal Navy as a career, I would still be greeted with the call of 'Er – Todd-boy – you still owe me for those wretched flannels', a reference to an aberrant fountain pen that had, many years before, ejected ink everywhere just before Joe decided to sit on my desk. Decades later, I still look carefully when wearing chinos before sitting down; I remain convinced he will one day take his revenge.

All this is a rather rambling diversion from the point that St Edward's set and marked not just the path for the next twenty years of my life but for how I both survived and rose above what I still consider a great wrong, born of lazy leadership and prejudice from people of whom I expected much better. So, after O levels in 1970, my term were all pushed to decide what A levels to subsequently pursue, and with only rudimentary career guidance, I succeeded in deciding that I either wanted to be a doctor or an engineer, and a naval one at that. Although I was unaware of it then, my father's father had been a naval officer (albeit that I may have been influenced too by two uncles, one still then serving – a redoubtable submariner and world record-setting deep-sea diver in the physical mould of James Robertson Justice meets Captain Birds Eye). In truth, as a small boy I had really wanted to be a Royal Marine but I reckon this may have been occasioned more by an attraction to their white pith helmets. Either way, a life in the Queen's Navy beckoned. First step was a three-day familiarisation trip to the Britannia Royal Naval College (BRNC) at Dartmouth, where I fell head over heels for the blond 'sea daddy' cadet assigned to look after me. I remember his name and that I kept an eye on his career for decades afterwards, but discretion precludes me from spilling the beans and, quite aside from (I hope) his never knowing the effect he had upon me, I'm not sure that our paths ever passed properly again. After this it was a race to join up: two days at the Admiralty Interview Board led to an offer to become a 'General List Engineer'. I could write pages about the Interview Board but 'tis better summarised by recalling a much-loved and well-known book called, with some originality, *We Joined the Navy* by the author and, later, obituarist John Winton that featured in its first chapter an hilarious account of the same Admiralty Interview Board at work and a grumble by the civilian headmaster on the Board to the effect that that day's candidates were all 'halfwits', causing the President to retort that this was quite alright as the Navy would add the other half in its own time and way.

So, before I knew it, I had completed my tenure at Teddies and was off – on a school trip (jointly with Harrow and Berkhamsted schools) to the Munich Olympic Games: a pre-Dartmouth indulgence by my parents that was memorable and tragic, in equal measure, for the excitement of the first of the really great modern Games and the tragedy of the massacre of eleven Israeli athletes and coaches and a West German police officer by Black September Palestinian terrorists. Our group had been quite privileged, partly as one of our party's father was the British team's senior doctor, which gave us good access, and that we were also guests of the Bavarian Youth Organisation, put up in a sixth-form school, fed by the German Army (breakfast) and the university (lunch and dinner). Most evenings, notwithstanding our ages, were spent in the famous Hofbräuhaus where, as soon as the Games' swimming and diving events were out of the way, we befriended the GB and Australian aquatic teams and became regular night-time revellers (and singers). So too, towards the end of the second week, did we find ourselves enlisted, like most of the youth of Munich, in putting tens of thousands of flags into mourning over one incredibly sad night, carefully draping or festooning every one with long black ribbons of commensurate size. Given the height of some of the flagpoles and the relative paucity of cherry pickers, I'm not sure how it was done safely and without injury, but it was.

A week later I was en route, courtesy of my father and the family Humber Sceptre (metallic gold with a black leatherette roof), albeit with me at the wheel, from Liverpool to Dartmouth, with an overnight stay in Dulverton, at Aunt Hillo's – although she wasn't actually an aunt but my father's cousin on his mother's side. I'd only passed my driving test scant months before – something that my father had accounted many years later to having surprised if not alarmed him as I'd shot straight onto a roundabout while driving to the test station, apparently right in front of another car that had had the good sense to brake quickly. However, at last my appointment with destiny and the Royal Navy was upon me; the day was Tuesday, 19 September 1972.

I and some hundred other midshipmen were to be the first of the new Naval College Entrant scheme, somewhat peeving for those who had already been at Dartmouth for one or two terms as cadets on the predecessor 'Murray' scheme, where the first year was normally spent as cadets before a second year as midshipmen undergoing sea training ('Fleet time') and then back to BRNC for a year of academic training as fledgling sub lieutenants. Finding themselves newly elevated to midshipmen alongside ourselves somewhat blunted their ability to lord it over us terrible new oiks.

Our first eight weeks were spent without any shore leave (i.e. freedom to head down after dinner to savour the many delights – mainly pubs – of Dartmouth) but, instead, being quickly broken down physically and mentally and reassembled, equally quickly, as young naval officers with a markedly different mindset and, too, vocabulary. Mornings started with 'Early Morning Activities' (EMAs) at 0600 sharp, which varied from a run to brass cannon cleaning to Morse code practice to four lengths of the swimming pool, most of this spent shivering in wait for one's turn. After a shower (luckily hot; the days of cold showers had, thankfully, been left well behind) and breakfast it was then time for 'After Breakfast Activities' (ABAs) at 0745, which varied between parade training with Divisions (the Navy's term for more formalised marching around, interspersed with prayers conducted by one of the chaplains, all ably assisted by the College's fine Royal Marine band) on Tuesdays and Thursdays, more Morse practice and a short talk in the College's main hall, the 'Sir Caspar John Hall', named after, for reasons that defy me, a rather po-faced past First Sea Lord and famous Fleet Air Arm aviator.

I remain quite astounded by how much was packed into those early weeks. Parade training dominated much at the outset and I recall the astonishment of the parade training staff (all GIs – Gunnery Instructors – aside from the Royal Marine colour sergeant ('Don't call me Colours, I'm not a bleedin' rainbow')) when they found that they had one of their own in our midst, now an 'Upper Yardman', i.e. someone promoted through the ranks while still in their teens or early twenties – young enough to be lumped in with the rest of us at BRNC (and I did warn about the rapidly changing vocabulary). Between ABAs and lunch (and with river activities taking up the brighter part of those afternoons that weren't spent on the playing fields) and dinner, we somehow crammed in eight lessons daily, including Navigation, Seamanship, Weapons Engineering, Mechanical Engineering, Operations (which I think then may have been called Warfare) and the delightfully named 'SAM' (Supply, Administration and Management). And then, too, there was introductory Meteorology, Oceanography, NBCD (Nuclear, Chemical, Biological Warfare and Damage Control), Aerodynamics and Ship Stability. And Communications, including more Morse.

Rounds. Not, as one might think, something one got caught for in the pub (although this was to come later, with a vengeance), but naval, for evening inspection. I was amazed some years later to discover that our Army colleagues at Sandhurst had nothing similar to contend with but, especially with us first-termers, Rounds stood for a right palaver with various duty personnel stomping around, much attempted blowing on a bosun's call, and woe betide anyone whose cabin (most of us were four to six to a cabin – what we previously might have called a shared bedroom, albeit with Navy issue steel bunks) didn't sparkle and gleam and whose boots and shoes weren't mirror-like. And that was before one's kit locker – a strange contraption, part wardrobe with sliding drawers to one side and surmounted by a boot rack – was inspected. As we'd found out fairly rapidly, every single bit of issued kit had a specific place of stowage. Each drawer was devoted to one type of clothing such as sports kit, where shorts and shirts, predictably four of each, two dark blue and two white, were required to be folded, to the nearest tenth of an inch, into perfect squares and then fitted into the drawers so they resembled a slice of blue and white Battenberg cake. I've never quite lost the inclination to fold shorts to this day into perfect squares. The more fastidious of us even invested in an additional set of most items so that we avoided constantly having to launder, fold and then iron back into position those that we used pretty much daily.

Some of us quickly developed the knack of 'bulling' our boots and black lace-up shoes to a state that would have made most guardsmen feel that they were somehow lacking – it really does take patience, spit and the best quality (and pre-washed) yellow duster that money can buy. And Kiwi black polish (all other brands being deemed inferior). I recall a Malaysian midshipman (we trained officers from many other navies in those days) once experimenting with linoleum polish, which quite outshone everyone for a while until it rained one Divisions and to the shock-horror of the GIs and to our delight, his parade boots started bubbling like a witch's cauldron, with the odd rainbow-hued bubble even floating away.

And, with my previous reference to the blond 'sea daddy' on my BRNC acclimatisation trip, some of you may by now have begun to wonder about the thought of nearly 500 young, fit men all rammed together, often in very close quarters. Were we actually human, with all the normal needs and wants of testosterone-loaded youths? Well, I suppose we must have been but aside from some minor flirting with the stout young ladies of Dartmouth (closely guarded and chaperoned by their male counterparts who we were forever being warned off getting into a fight with), and the appearance of 'girl friends' from back home at the end of term Ball (I was paired off with the Commander's daughter, an attractive but disinterested and dull girl with whom I was obviously on very careful alert lest her father received a dubious report), it was as if sex, let alone sexuality, did not exist. I wouldn't say that we were modest – it's very difficult when fifty of you are trying to get through ten showers all at the same time following afternoon sport – but I always kept my eyes carefully averted. My latter two years at Teddies had produced some regular 'fun' with a couple of friends, but discretely. If the hotbed of tortured public school sin and depravity ever existed, I, alas, never found it. So it was too at Dartmouth and, with virtually no exceptions, for the entirety of my naval career.

Lieutenant Patrick Lyster-Todd, Executive Officer HMS *Alert*, Northern Ireland, 1979.

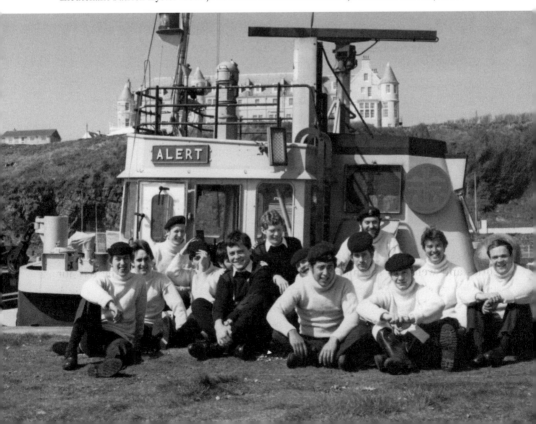

Fairly early on – after waking one morning in a strange bed with the smell of freshly ground coffee and the previous night's 'pick-up' from the vast public gents at Waterloo station preparing breakfast while I was directed to the wardrobe for a spare dressing gown, thereupon gazing upon two policemen's helmets neatly side by side – I had evolved my Rules. These enabled me to 'survive' in the Navy while also being able to take into account my proclivity for playing the 'pink oboe' and, preferably, someone else's: firstly, there were to be no boyfriends and also no gay friends and, definitely, no sex with other uniformed personnel. I could, however, if I judged it to be sufficiently at arm's length, have physical 'liaisons' – but never the same guy for more than, if I was lucky, a single weekend.

These were good rules: good in the sense that I was able to have my cake and eat it, to develop a long service career in the Royal Navy, to aspire one day to command of one of Her Majesty's warships but not to go fully mad from denying myself the pleasures of Eros. I went through the rest of my teens, all my twenties and well into my thirties this way: never a partner, never a close friend who really knew who I was. Never to fall in love – although, of that, I'm not so sure. I met many fabulous, gorgeous young men over the years, no small number of whom I'd have loved to have met again. With very few exceptions and those in the last half decade, I never did. I often accepted a scribbled address or telephone number (no mobile phones or internet in those days) and I developed the knack of always tearing up these scraps of paper and scattering them through the train window en route back to whatever port and ship I was serving in; more latterly, through car windows. I didn't really think too much of it at the time – but every time I did this, a part of me died. Life was not allowed to be 'normal': this was just how it was and I had to get on with it, always being my own counsel.

Nor could I afford to buy anything that marked me as who I really was – none of the early gay magazines or papers. I learnt, usually when I was up in London on my own for a weekend, to 'find' where other people like me congregated. In the early to mid-1970s we were less than a decade since the 1967 Sexual Offences Act finally made homosexuality legal in England and Wales (only), provided you were over 21 and only had sex in private (that did not include a hotel room nor the presence of anyone else). Significantly, the new Act did not extend to members of Her Majesty's Armed Forces (or, then, Merchant Navy). It was to take decades before a semblance of equality and acceptance was to emerge in British society generally and the fight (for that was what it was for those of us who campaigned for change) is still far from over even today in 2019. Back then, in the seventies, eighties and well into the nineties, circumspection was the order of the day for many who were attracted to the same sex. Many developed and lived two entirely separate lives although, slowly, people started to assert themselves. Barely months before I joined the Navy, the UK's first Pride march was held in London on 1 July 1972 (chosen as the nearest Saturday to the anniversary of the New York Stonewall

Inn riots of 28 June 1969, where a small group of the gay and trans community spontaneously stood up to a heavy-handed police raid, giving rise to the birth of the Pride movement and to LGBTQ people first campaigning for themselves and their own rights), which attracted approximately 2,000 participants.

I tore up that very first slip from my Saturday night policeman (containing his address and telephone number) and although I managed to get both of the subsequent weekends off and spent each desperately searching for his flat, somewhere in the Kennington area, I was never to find it. I sometimes wonder what might have happened if we'd met again – whether life and my career might have turned out entirely differently. It was not to be.

In the years and decades that ensued, I continued to live my rather odd double life. From time to time there was a girlfriend and it would be entirely wrong to infer that I didn't sometimes enjoy these relatively short periods. In one sense, they helped maintain the pretence of being a professional bachelor officer. As my positions and responsibilities grew with experience, I soon found that I needed to be, as it was then known, 'Positively Vetted' in order to allow me access to secret materials – top secret in some instances, with additional levels of access and clearance applied over this too. Vetting then, as now, was largely a process of determining beyond reasonable doubt or risk that an individual could be entrusted with the nation's most sensitive or secret information and, above all, that they were beyond any possibility of blackmail or coercion. I had to prepare myself for my first vetting interview, which was conducted by an exceptionally straight-faced, moustached and humourless retired Royal Marine major. Having decided that honesty – or, at least, the truth, if not necessarily the whole truth – was the line to take, it was with some trepidation that we reached the 'homosexuality questions', as I had come to anticipate them.

'Have you ever had any homosexual thoughts or a homosexual experience?' To which I had, rather convincingly I believed, squirmed on my seat and confessed that while at school there had been some thoughts and a few furtive fumbles. Leading me on helpfully, he then asked if these were just the normal thoughts that a fit young man going through puberty and the period afterwards might have, to which I had wholeheartedly agreed, to whit that my thoughts were indeed nothing more than that. 'Nothing, er ... ever *came out*, did it?' Not entirely sure what exactly he might be referring to, I ventured a confident and slightly wounded 'certainly not', which met with approval. He continued ... 'And have you had any other experience of this – er – behaviour – since?' I took a deep breath and recounted the story, from four or five years before when I had been on my midshipmen's training cruise in the Caribbean on board the assault ship HMS *Intrepid* and when, on returning late from drinking ashore with fellow midshipmen, I had found myself in the company of one of our embarked helicopter pilots, a young Royal Marine lieutenant, who subsequently offered to show me the flight and aircrew offices and briefing room. It was somewhere well past midnight, I had still

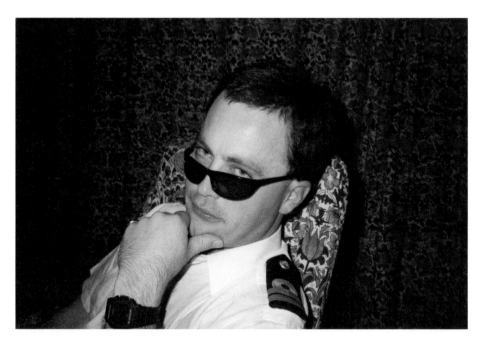

Bachelor and man about town.

to turn 18 and was quite inebriated, but nevertheless went along with this unlikely diversion. No sooner than being safely secreted in the briefing room did I realise that I was being presented with a rather toothy smile, a large and gently nodding member and something about whether I would like to say hello to 'Mr Proddy', this being, I should add, before I had even heard of Roger Hargreaves and his Mr Men. 'Good grief,' interjected my vetting officer, 'what happened then?' The truth of the matter was that I was in a bit of a dilemma – but, bodily functions to the fore, I said, 'Well, I was sick.' Which I was, all over the floor of the briefing room – disappearing, soon afterwards, to leave Mr Proddy to clear it all up. 'Good chap – I'm not surprised,' said the Royal Marine major before, satisfied that I was as heterosexual as they came, moving on to questions about my back account.

I was to face vetting again some ten years later when it came up for review, and at that time I had the somewhat grandiose title of Staff Operations Officer (Surface and Air) at the Clyde Submarine Base at Faslane in Dunbartonshire; it abbreviated nicely to SOO(SA) to COMCLYDENORLANT (which, for the uninitiated, stood for Commodore Clyde, North Atlantic Command). Somewhere I still have my NATO badge. My job, along with my opposite number, Staff Operations Officer (Submarines) or SOO(SM), was to run the operations room and be responsible (Royal Marine Commachio Company notwithstanding) for the broader surface and air defence of the National Deterrent. For those who can remember James Bond's *The Spy Who Loved Me*, our operations room actually

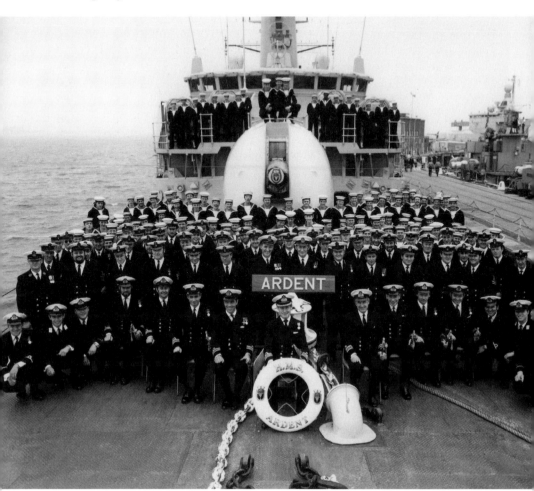

The Ship's Company, HMS *Ardent*, 1978. I am third from the left on the front row. *Ardent* was lost in San Carlos Water on 21 May 1982. Her subsequent commanding officer was Commander Alan West DSC, an officer who later became First Sea Lord and a strong advocate for equality.

featured in the film, although, to be honest, it wasn't the same one. The one in the film featured an elaborate and carefully guarded Top Secret display that ostensibly showed the location of the 'on patrol' nuclear deterrent submarine. In fact, I recall that it actually disappeared off the screen at the critical moment, swallowed up by some monster tanker. The reality was somewhat more prosaic, with the location of the same submarine easily calculated from a pencilled line on a rolled-up chart in the bottom of the 10th Submarine Squadron's Operations Officer's cabinet safe. In those days we put more trust in a 2B pencil and one of Her Majesty's Hydrographic Office's finest but he had great fun showing it to those very few of us who were entitled. The film had appeared some ten years before.

But back to my vetting review, having set the scene. At that time a good number of those based at Faslane would head south for the weekend, booking their flights through the redoubtable Murray & Biggar Travel Agency in nearby Helensburgh. And there worked the apple of every sailor's and officer's eye from miles around: the gorgeous, leggy blonde – let us call her Susan. I daresay that many a sailor or wayward lieutenant booked all manner of unwanted trips and holidays for no reason other than that, with careful timing, they could be served by the lovely and wholly not innocent Susan. So, as a bachelor (and fairly fit in those days) lieutenant commander, with my own pad overlooking Rhu Narrows, the entrance to the Gare Loch and Faslane, and with lashings of charm and guile, I became the envy and voodoo pin puppet for most of the wardroom and ship's company at the base. My reputation had obviously preceded or, at least, intercepted the visiting vetting officer, who completely passed over any questions about homosexuality in favour of picking my finances apart (I'd recently rather over-extended myself in buying a fabulous new house in Southsea, some 500 miles away).

I had by now spent sixteen years in the Navy, become a middle-ranking officer with a more focused eye on aspiring to what is quaintly known as a 'brass hat', viz. a cap with 'scrambled egg' or, more accurately, gold wire 'oak leaf sprig' embellishment denoting a senior officer and, most important of all, command of my own frigate or destroyer. And, in all those years, from naïf to worldly man, I had never had a proper partner – just a few 'girl friends' who maintained the James Bond appearance of someone not built for settling down and producing a brood of ankle-biters. I was very much by no means a saint – but I craved some permanence in my life and it was to be forever denied to me: 'like it or lump it', as the saying went. My evenings and leave periods ran the risk of being sad and lonely but, luckily, I did have one other thing going for me – and that was that I was also a maverick and extrovert. When younger I had sometimes been accused of being naïve; in fact, I'd even been put on a month's official warning for this during my midshipmen's cruise on board HMS *Intrepid*. Perhaps I *was* naïve but I preferred to consider myself as cut from slightly different cloth, which, of course, I was, but then I was hardly going to admit to gold lamé and sequins. One of the manifestations of all of this, from the late 1970s until the early 1990s, was my proclivity for Club 18-30 holidays where I could really be myself and had also, discretely, learned that a good 25 per cent of fit young straight Brits on holiday, especially when faced with the prospect of returning to their hotels and Portland Villa apartments in the early hours without having succeeded in getting 'their leg over', might very well succumb to my masculine charms as a satisfactory and harmless alternative. I recall that some used to come back for seconds too.

For anyone else, going on an 18-30 holiday was definitely *not* officer territory – but then there was no law about it and I cultivated such wayward behaviour as being part of my free spirit and extrovertism. In reality, all my brother officers

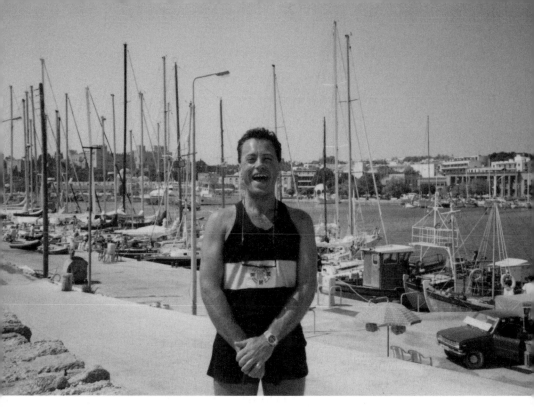

The Club 18-30 Patrick Lyster-Todd, 'fun in the sun'.

would normally hang on to my every word when I debriefed after returning from two weeks in Corfu or Palma Nova or San Antonio. The holiday snaps, quickly checked in advance by myself, were awaited with glee and some envy.

And while on my 18-30 adventures, I did learn to play a different role: still ostensibly a 'straight' man, I would normally assume the role of a sailor or, to be more precise, a senior rating – invariably, as I got older, as a petty officer or chief petty officer. In those days a good fifth of all 18-30 holiday-goers were serving military (something, I suspect, that the Ministry of Defence had never cottoned on to, not that it really mattered) so to be able to integrate on these fun-filled excursions, it was very wise not to present as an officer. And the strange thing was that within a few days of arrival in a resort, a 'team' of mainly other servicemen would have gravitated to my orbit and would look to me for their lead. It was a lot of fun and I learnt never to leave my camera unattended when it was my round by the pool in the evening. I'm not necessarily saying that any had detected the possibility that I might bat for the other side but I certainly accumulated some rather interesting and unexpected pictures over the years (Boots would position a strategically placed adhesive sticker over any offending shots, although these could usually be peeled off without metaphoric castration).

One balmy evening in early June 1988 at Faslane, I therefore held my annual 'SOO(SA) Club 18-30 Pre-Tenerife Party' at my apartment – Hawaiian shirts and shorts compulsory – and welcomed in friends and colleagues from the Operations

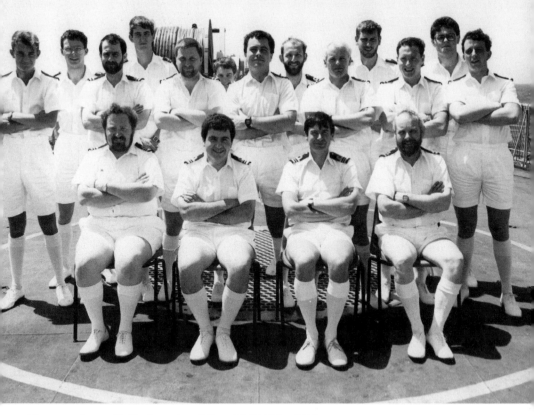

Lieutenant Lyster-Todd, Operations Officer HMS *Sirius*, 1986.

team to other submarine squadrons, with COMCLYDE himself and wife, as ever, wearing one of the more outrageous outfits. We all had a marvellous time, laughed and danced and drank far too much. Yet, on this occasion, I was not to make it to the fleshpots of Playa de las Américas in Tenerife and, within a week, was in intensive care in partial isolation at Ruchill NHS Hospital in Glasgow.

When I say that I tended to do things that others might find a little odd, this extended to the game of paintball where I had risen to the dizzy heights of being Captain of the Scottish Champions, the 'Team With No Name' (mainly as we couldn't agree on one; it later became 'Team Highlander', of even greater fame). Paintball, for the uninitiated, consists of two teams of some dozen players each who both charge around a variety of different natural or artificial settings and generally try to shoot the heck out of one another with coloured paintballs fired from some very hi-tech and SF-esque compressed-air guns. One price frequently paid, especially if caught reversing out of some inoffensive rhododendron bush, was the tendency to acquire multiple and beautifully hued bruises in strange and exciting parts of one's anatomy. And, for some months now, I had been complaining to the base doctors of a strange ache down my right-hand side, especially below my right ribcage. Naturally it was ascribed to paintball war injuries, but I was slowly becoming aware of other symptoms: dark urine and very pale number twos. Within three days of the party, from which I had been very slow – unusually for me – to recover, wandering around in a bit of a daze for much of the Sunday, not being able to put my finger on why I felt so tired and lethargic, the whites of my eyes had turned AA-yellow, my father had driven up from Liverpool and I knew that I had hepatitis. After a very difficult night in my apartment, I was reduced to crawling … and by 8 am in the morning, an ambulance arrived to cart me off. I had hepatitis B and, it later transpired, 95 per cent liver failure.

Amazingly, I pulled through within a fortnight while the NHS and the Navy looked hard for an O rhesus negative transplant liver; even the United States Navy was roped in but, luckily, it was not needed – which was just as well as they didn't locate one. I learnt that hepatitis B was a notifiable disease (unlike HIV, which had just started to strike heavily within the gay community in London), requiring sexual partner tracing – which placed me in a difficult situation, partly alleviated by not knowing who any of my periodic partners were (this being, thankfully, before the lovely Susan). In truth, it later transpired that I had probably caught it when helping out at a road traffic accident in Edinburgh when a student had been knocked over by a motorcyclist. After stopping the traffic, ascertaining that the motorcyclist was alright, if winded and bruised, and having allocated various tasks to passers-by and motorists who had stopped to assist, I was called across to the student, lying in a pool of blood, in shock and with his right tibia protruding through his jeans. The blood was from a head wound, quickly staunched, but I needed to check, without moving him, that he wasn't bleeding elsewhere. I grazed the backs of both hands on the road surface and, well … that was that. The student survived and, probably, benefitted too from being told subsequently that he also had hepatitis B. Luckily, as it later turned out, that was all he had.

Recuperation required an extended period of convalescence – taken at my parents' home in Liverpool where, conveniently, our next-door neighbour was Professor of Medical Microbiology at Liverpool's main teaching hospital and a leading expert in viro-immunology. So I found myself in good hands and recovered far more rapidly than had been anticipated. It was during one of my subsequent visits down to my new home in Southsea and a Sunday afternoon foray to a gay sauna in Rottingdean that I met someone who was to change my life for ever. His name was Dennis and he was 27 (I was 33) and, like so many other similar encounters in the past, we ended up exchanging telephone numbers in the car park afterwards. However, after placing this in my wallet, a torrential downpour opened up and, with windows remaining firmly closed on a focused drive back on the A27 to Southsea, I forgot about it.

By now, I was fit enough to return to work at Faslane. It was on my first trip back to Southsea, for a long weekend, some months later that I rediscovered the note – a yellow Post-it – tucked away in my wallet while on my BMI flight to

Heathrow. And I very much remembered Dennis: slim, blondish, not classically good-looking – but, to me, extremely attractive. And he was happily out, balanced, sorted, funny. What to lose from giving him a call? We agreed to meet that same weekend, in Croydon, where he lived in the family home – parents Barbara and Dennis senior away for several months in the South of France – and never looked back.

Slowly, deliciously, I fell in love for the first time in my life and to hell with the Rules. I still had just under a year in Faslane but a long-distance relationship was just fine and relatively easy to manage. Moving back down to Southsea the next year, in a way, just made it even better. I'd acquired yet another well-regarded appointment – as Head of Junior Officers' Training at the School of Maritime Operations, HMS Dryad, in the delightful, feudal village of Southwick, just north of Portsmouth, responsible for the famed 'Officer of the Watch' course and all other tertiary operations training for young officers returning from Fleet time.

The commute between Southsea and Croydon took just over an hour but ensured sufficient distance when staying in Croydon to not have to look too closely over my shoulder. Yet my home in Southsea (part of a Grade II listed converted

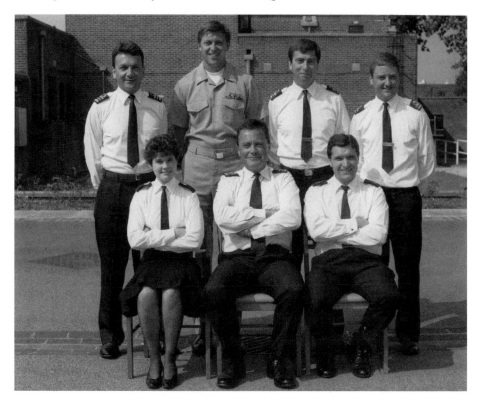

The new 'Staff Officer Junior Officer Training', HMS Dryad, 1991.

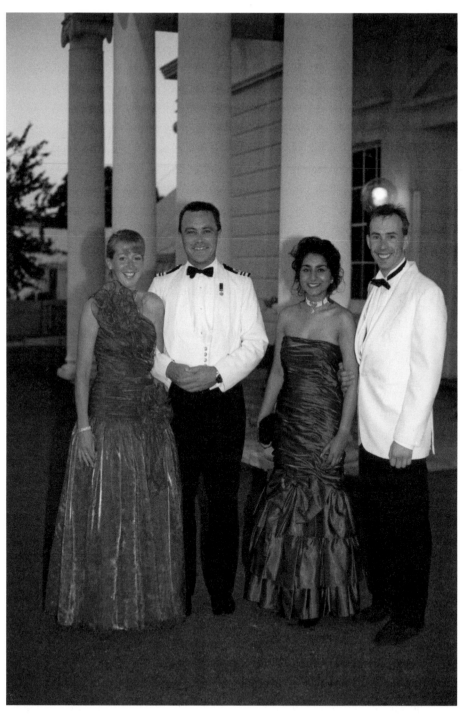

Dennis and me, pictured with 'girlfriends', HMS Dryad, summer ball, 1991.

Victorian convent with a spiral wooden staircase from the vaulted chapel ceiling of the living room down to two enormous bedrooms) became *our* home and this required some careful planning, especially as a couple of other naval officers had apartments – luckily some distance away – within the complex.

With our joint incomes we could afford to holiday regularly and the ability to travel somewhere where no one really cared who we were or even if we were a same-sex couple – even back then as we turned from the 1980s to the 1990s – with some circumspection meant that we could keep our life separated from my naval one.

I had, however, noticed when rummaging for some socks back in Croydon one Friday afternoon (Dennis was working late) an amazing array of pills, capsules and tablets secreted away in his bedroom chest of drawers. Most of them I'd never heard of before – Trimethoprim (and Bactrim), Zovirax and others. One unmarked bottle held a large number of white capsules with a central blue band. It was quite mystifying. In the end, I drew a little diagram of each one and several days later, having taken the afternoon off, found myself sitting in the reference section of Portsmouth City Library with a copy of the British National Formulary in front of me. Eventually, I had them all identified aside from the blue-banded capsule, yet I still couldn't really work out what all these drugs meant. About to give up for the moment, I flicked through the index at the rear of the BNF ... and an addendum fell out. Within this, I finally identified Azidothymidine (or Zidovudine). My heart sank as I read, 'An experimental drug used in the treatment of the retrovirus, Human Immunodeficiency Virus or HIV'.

Dennis was HIV positive.

We were not due to meet for several days and I just had to speak. Perhaps unkindly, I telephoned him that night and revealed what I had discovered. There was a very long pause when all I could hear was his breathing over the phone. 'Do you want to end it?' he asked very quietly.

With tears in my eyes, I replied gently, 'You silly little sausage. Of course not.'

He drove down that night (and we both called in sick the following morning – something I had never faked before, but to hell with it) and we talked for ages, until we fell into bed and slept a dreamless sleep in one another's arms. He told me that the last two guys he'd dated had both dropped him when he'd told them about his status.

The years slipped by and the nineties arrived. By this stage I'd made myself a bit of an expert on HIV and AIDS – but it was never really a topic that we discussed in depth. We both knew that the horizon, for the moment, was clear, but beyond lurked an iceberg and, actually, perhaps it was better not to know how far beyond it floated.

I enjoyed my new job enormously. I had a good team and the ability to make a difference, and together with my staff drove through some important changes,

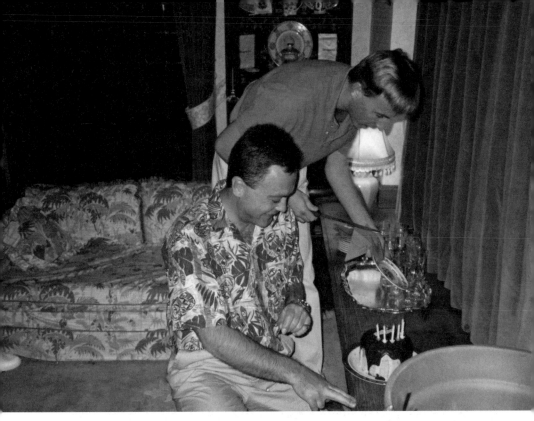
A treasured memory of a very happy birthday with Dennis, 1989.

not least in preparing for the introduction of the Navy's first full bridge simulator, redesign of the main Officer of the Watch course and rationalisation of the course's annual prizes. Ship Command exams – essential if I wanted to aspire to Command – started to assume more priority and my Appointer, responsible for deciding upon my next job, let slip that I could expect to be appointed as the First Lieutenant (and second-in-command) of one of our fourteen Type 42 guided-missile destroyers. Dennis continued well – but with some minor health niggles: stomach upsets, periodic tiredness – nothing serious but, occasionally, enough to make me think about our future. Slowly, I came to the realisation that there was no way that I could allow myself to be deployed with my next warship, possibly halfway around the world, only for Dennis to fall ill and need me. For sure the Navy would do everything it could to get me home to my partner and, too, I could envisage my commanding officer asking me if I knew what might be wrong with her as we diverted to get me to the nearest main airport, our helicopter pilot busily calculating just how soon he could get airborne to meet whatever flight was being held for me. And I would have had to reply that it was not a 'her' but a 'him'.

I'd still be despatched home – but this time to be met by two provost marshals of the same rank as myself – and to be placed under open arrest, to await my inevitable court martial for … being who I was. The maximum sentence, occasionally used, was two years in detention at the Army's Military Corrective Training Centre in Colchester. In truth, I'd probably just be chucked out, but Colchester remained an option and, for an officer, that meant virtual solitary confinement. I just couldn't do it – not to myself or to my family, to my parents who were proud of my military service (my father was a retired army colonel and my mother a wartime WAAF officer – at least until my sister came along) but, especially, not to Dennis. So, after a short period of research, I chose to voluntarily resign early.

Everyone, not least my boss, thought I was mad. 'Why?' they asked – you're doing well; get the next job right and you'll have your brass hat. Well, I assembled some rather unconvincing but resolute story that I wanted to get out so I could establish a new career elsewhere while young enough. Some, I suspect, asked themselves what the real reason was – but people did do strange things and there was no reason why I couldn't be as strange as they. I was required to give a year's notice (by way of 'return of service', i.e. as part-payment for all that had been lavished on and invested in me to get me where I was). I was extended in my current position as Staff Officer Junior Officers' Training, which would

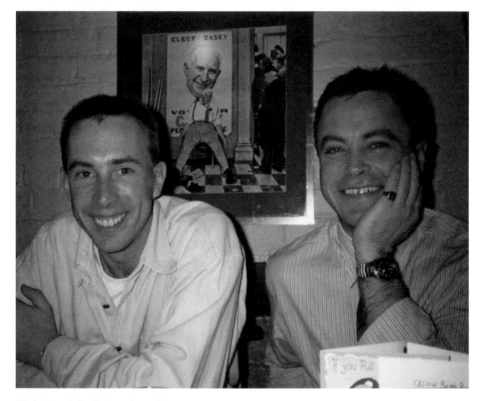

With Dennis in the happiest of times.

now be my last and, luckily, it was also agreed that my last official day for pay would be a couple of weeks past my thirty-seventh birthday, thus securing a good resettlement package ('golden handshake') plus just hooking an immediate pension – although I commuted most of this for fifteen years to secure an additional lump sum.

Early in 1992, Dennis spent a couple of days in hospital for the first time – nothing that could be identified in particular, except that he just felt absolutely wasted. He recovered quickly but, for both of us, it was a wake-up call that, AZT and several prophylactic drugs notwithstanding (these often being taken by those who were HIV positive but asymptomatic to ward off certain AIDS-defining illnesses), there was still absolutely no cure, nor sight of one, nor anything that could really keep, unlike today, the virus suppressed so that it caused little damage to the body's immune system.

As my departure from the Navy approached, we made plans for life after: a big holiday out to the Far East plus buying a small flat in London, which required shopping lists and colour schemes and much else.

I also debated the possibility of starting up my own business as a franchisee with an American importer called, somewhat conveniently, 'Decorating Den's'. We never found out who 'Den' was and, frankly, I'm glad it never came to be as it never took off as a franchise operation. I would have been a glorified Avon Lady, harking my wares and somewhat dubious soft-furnishing and decorating ideas around in a gaudy van to unsuspecting, bored ladies who would be provided to me as 'leads', no doubt cultivated from the back pages of *The Lady* and *Country Life*. Dennis and I invented a range of new colours for the latter such as 'Dead Rabbit', 'Labrador Yellow' and 'Parson Puce', but I reckoned that he was more worried that I might succumb to the charms and Victoria sponge cake of one of the aforementioned ladies. With some irony, my great straight friend – one of my very few, harking back to university days in Newcastle (during a sojourn from the Navy) – happened upon a restaurant franchise called 'Pierre Victoire', setting up one such establishment overlooking the weir in the beautiful town of Bath. Not that many years later, I followed, albeit as a company man, to take over Bristol's Pierre Victoire restaurant. But all that is for a rainy day.

As the daffodils started to appear in spring 1992, Dennis began to deteriorate. These days, daffodils always hold a special meaning. Dennis would probably say this was because they were cheap but, for me, they always marked a sense of renewal … of coming spring – a brash and colourful prelude on the heels of the snowdrops and crocuses before the rainbow arrival of the first tulips. Healthwise, it was nothing that one could really put one's finger on: just an increasing general malaise that forebode ill and that both of us nevertheless took in our stride and didn't linger over too much. Easy for me. Then, somewhat suddenly, when down in Southsea for a weekend approaching mid-March, he declared on the Sunday morning that he felt he needed to be back in hospital. Dennis senior drove down quickly and within hours, Dennis junior had been admitted to Charing Cross Hospital (slightly confusingly in Hammersmith).

He was never to leave.

Days became weeks and, successively, he fought off one opportunistic infection after another. His immune system had collapsed totally, as had his platelet count, which probably explained the constant tiredness and proclivity to bruise easily. I took to travelling up every other early evening, staying with him in his single room on the hospital's main cardiac ward where he had been placed and then driving back to be home by midnight and up again at 6 am. Life almost became normalised and I became a known and regular visitor by Dennis's bedside. His greatest pleasure lay in having a warm bath, which I would take charge of, kneeling by the side, gently sponging him and making unhelpful comments about feeling horny. In truth, anything to turn a smile – which came readily, though from what depth of reserve I had no idea.

Looking back on those days, one of the things I remember most about Dennis is the bravery with which he faced the only outcome open to him then: stoic, uncomplaining, courageous to the end. On his last Sunday, sat on the bed in his hospital room with one arm wrapped gently around him while the other held a kidney dish into which he retched up the most vile yellow liquid, I was not to know that this was to be the last time we would ever sit together as a pair – as partners and lovers, confidantes and best friends; soulmates. All, of course, a secret to my employers, for whom all this on my part was a criminal act.

This following week was to be my last in the Royal Navy and, unlike in previous weeks, I was not going to be able to drive up to London from Portsmouth every other day to spend my few hours with Dennis and relieve his parents and brother on their own vigil. Ironically, of course, that was indeed just what I did do on the Wednesday evening, phoned by his mother within minutes of a sudden cardiac arrest and of the consultants deciding, so rightly, not to attempt resuscitation.

He was still warm when I arrived, barely two hours later – with his hair neatly brushed, a fresh white T-shirt on, bathed just in the soft light from above the washbasin in the adjoining private lavatory, the door barely ajar: as handsome as ever I remember him, at peace, looking like the beautiful young god that, to me, he had always been.

I had, with some prescience, pre-laid an excuse with my boss that a very close friend was critically ill, so when I phoned asking for the following day off – my final Thursday – it was approved swiftly. Just as well, as I had to engineer getting his parents and younger brother home to Croydon later that night where, fortified with considerable cognac, I slept not a wink and watched with great disinterest the only thing on the television – the General Election results when Prime Minister Major somewhat unexpectedly found himself returned to No. 10.

The immediate aftermath of Dennis's death was, mercifully, taken up with matters of necessity and my twenty years' military training fired up well. That Thursday was my own 'longest day', starting with a return trip to the hospital with Dennis's parents, plotted carefully via known ladies' loos as his mother, Barbara, could barely survive for more than twenty minutes. There was much paperwork at the hospital, an offer to see him again (politely declined – we had all said our goodbyes the previous night) and, for me, a very useful conversation in private with one of the two doctors on duty the previous day who had rushed to his side, shooing his mother out, when he had arrested. Being on the cardiac ward, immediately next door to the coronary care unit – well, yes, they probably could have restarted him with a reasonable chance of success, but they chose not to (we didn't, quite, have Advance Decisions in those days): he would, almost certainly, have faced little more than seventy-two hours, invariably on some form of intubation and with no doubt whatsoever in his own mind about what was fast approaching. They made, of course, the right decision and, in some small way, I think the junior consultant was reassured by my agreement and thanks that following morning. Thereafter, a trip to Fulham Town Hall to obtain the death certificate and copies, back home, via a trail of loos, for lunch, an appointment (for his father and myself) at the family funeral directors in Croydon where everything down to coffin trim was decided upon – and then, picking up Barbara en route, to the local vicar for tea and decisions over hymns. Back home again and on to the telephone calls: nearly 100 for me and about half that for Dennis senior. I cannot ever recall having to be so strong and brave, though I say it myself. I was faced with incredulity, tears, more heartbreak and the growing realisation that I was going to have to be strong for many days to come, for other people – let alone myself.

Finally, I was driven back home in my car to Portsmouth by Dennis's brother, Michael – late that first night (he just managing to catch the last train back to London) so that, the following morning, I could arrive into work at HMS Dryad and the Junior Officers' Section fresh and ready to hand over my department to my successor (my deputy), and, later, to host my leaving party for some 100, from the Commander-in-Chief Naval Home Command – Admiral Sir Jeremy Black, Chair of the Saint Barbara Association, of which I had until days before been the Secretary – to my own staff. I served Harvey Wallbangers and White Russians and took a taxi home, returning to pick up my car the following morning. This was one day I have never forgotten: I had woken abruptly, alone, in our bed in Southsea, and it had slowly dawned on me that the only two things that had ever truly mattered in my life had gone within the space of just forty-eight hours.

I spent much of the next month with Dennis's parents in south Croydon. There seemed plenty to keep us occupied until the funeral when, on the eve before, I realised that no one was attending from my own family. A very unsettling phone call ensued with my brother, and I was pleased enormously in consequence to see my own dear parents and sister-in-law at the crematorium the following lunchtime – my brother, alas, having a meeting that he just could not extricate himself from. We had two wakes – one, more family-orientated back at his parents' and, once tea and sandwiches and respectable quantities of whisky had flowed, a second one at our great friends Mel and Fonz's mansion home on the heights of Kenley, along with all our gay friends. In many ways it was surreal, crowded around a roaring fire in the drawing room, lit by candles and one sidelamp, all our friends around – all but my one great friend, my first best friend and soulmate.

The days following were wholly anti-climactic with little to do and all the great plans that Dennis and I had been making, as recently as the month before, now laid to waste; even the holiday I'd booked half a year before – five weeks out to Thailand, Singapore, Bali and Hong Kong – all but forgotten. I'd given the operators, Thomas Cook, for whom Dennis had worked in medical repatriation, a telephone call to cancel the holiday but without any hope of even receiving a penny's worth of compensation for myself. Dennis had had a known condition and I, of course, might have anticipated such an outcome. No insurance policy would have covered either of us. To rather rub it in, they did offer to waive the standard charge of changing Dennis's name on the travel documentation lest I wanted to take someone else in his stead. I had one of my better moments in days when I'd told them where they could stick our holiday. I never heard from them again. £4000+ for the holiday of a lifetime was quite a bit for 1992 and I often wondered who in Thomas Cook benefitted the most; no doubt their shareholders. I have shunned them ever since.

I began to slide. Our home in Southsea, let alone anything to do with the Navy, was also forgotten and I spent most days wandering aimlessly around Croydon shopping centre, finding myself retracing the steps that, once, we'd taken between this shop and that restaurant, this store and that. And, returning back to south Croydon one early afternoon, to sit with Dennis senior as we always did, around the dining room table, tea and ashtray at hand, the dam finally broke. All that coping and being strong and organising, all those telephone calls and letters, all the weight of my long Jekyll & Hyde existence, the years of living two lives, of being lonely, of being committed to my naval life but of not having a proper bedrock emotionally, except for what I could create myself or else snatch at here and there and, since the arrival of Dennis, at least with some semblance of normality. That was, at least, if you forget the sword that wavered over our heads in terms of the virus, or of constantly looking over my shoulder, metaphorically or not, of always sitting in those restaurants in Portsmouth or Southsea when together, me facing the entrance so that I could quickly put on the face of dining with a friend should a naval acquaintance come in … suddenly all came to a single point of focus.

Dennis Senior, sensing that something was about to happen, quickly crossed to where I sat and there held me, in his arms, rocking me while I wept for some ten minutes – while I let everything out, all the pain and loss, the grief and disappointment, the hurt, frustrations, disbelief … and anger: that, in this 1990s Britain with all its tradition of decency, and democracy, of charity and kindness – of intellect and reason, that something like this could still occur – where a lifetime worked to date – *my* career – carried with dedication and a preparedness to, if necessary, lay down my life for my fellow colleague or countryman – counted for nothing. Not for me the support or sympathy or understanding when the person I loved had died.

That, in many ways, was the end of that life; thirty-seven years lived – and the twenty-seven years since – mark an entirely different journey, one that I could never have anticipated, where I both soared to unlikely heights and yet also, at times, was incredibly difficult and lonely, certainly sufficient for a psychiatrist to keep themselves well employed for years, probably ungainfully. It was, too, to be a new adventure and challenge, and that story is for telling in full another time, although you will find parts told elsewhere in this book by several other colleagues and good friends from those days. However, when I look back at this time, I sometimes ask myself if I have regrets and, of course, I do, but life marches forward and, to paraphrase some half-remembered quotation, 'once when time has writ its tale and moved on, not even Ozymandias and all his kings can call it back to change but a second of it'. That Dennis will now always be part of me casts all such regrets into shadow. That he inspired me to have a role in ensuring that, one day, men and women such as me, committed to the military but born to love those of the same sex, could serve without having to keep one eye perpetually cast over one's shoulder is a matter of great pride.

However, it would be wrong to suppose that this was a full turning point: it wasn't, and the new road ahead would still lead to several dead ends and many disappointments – but, for now, I had some sense of direction. Soon, therefore, I returned to Portsmouth – to pick up my life and wonder about my future.

Workwise, it was to be almost another three years before I returned to full-time employment – to be the new Health Promotion Officer for Positive People at the country's main HIV and AIDS charity, the Terrence Higgins Trust. I wasn't positive myself – which, in the most ridiculous of ways, later worked against me when it slowly became apparent that some of my new colleagues – never to my face and invariably through underhand comment or insinuation – wished that I was, in the sense that how on earth could I undertake this role effectively without the perspective that this would surely have brought. However, in that time I set the baseline for much that I would go on to undertake and achieve in the decades ahead – working in ways that I could not have foreseen both once again with the great military family and the voluntary, charitable sector – as well as in the hospitality field, both as restaurateur and licensee. In some ways, when measured over the years, it seemed that there was little that I could not turn my hand to successfully, but nothing really endured and I would soon find myself at yet another pinnacle before moving on.

With the benefit of experience and years, I have long since realised that I was still seeking what I had once had – a career embedded with the military and a partner who wanted to be with me and with whom I could spend the rest of my life. I had found it – and him – rather late in life when measured against my contemporaries – and, too, without some of the benefits that might have accrued in a more liberated and understanding time. Today, my husband and I – for I found again – have a good life. However, he knows too that not a day goes by that I do not still think of his predecessor and, in some way, I hope that he looks upon Dennis as an older brother whose path never crossed with his own.

Nevertheless, in the months after Dennis's death, I still had to regroup and establish what my new opportunities might be. I had money – a sizeable resettlement grant (accrued through serving sixteen years from the age of 21) which I had almost doubled by commuting – as one could then – the maximum amount allowed from my future pension. And I had no idea what I wanted to do now, especially without Dennis by my side to advise and assist me, no matter how long we might have had together. In fact, we'd always assumed that it would be a good few years. He had seemed well until the last six months of his life and, with my departure from the Navy looming large, had reckoned that with his salary, a presumed new one on my part, income from a flatmate in Southsea plus my resettlement monies, we could buy a small one-bedroomed flat somewhere in south London while also holding on to our main home as a future investment.

Early on, I was undoubtedly lethargic. I had a lovely home and days became lazy and somewhat indolent. Nor was I feeling that well, physically: minute, tiny clear blisters had started to form along the fine creases of both palms and I perpetually had the runs. Not badly – but consistently enough to worry me. When I started to sense minor paralysis in first my right hand and lower arm, and then my left one too, I realised that something was not right. Yet my GP was equally perplexed, especially as there was, despite a barrage of tests, nothing identifiably wrong with me. Eventually my symptoms were deemed psychosomatic: in short, brought about entirely by stress and anxiety – for Dennis, for the past risk of being discovered, and for the well of grief into which I had fallen. My best solution was, apparently, to take a holiday.

So it was that I booked myself, in late June 1992, to three weeks in Gran Canaria; to what became – and to this day remains – my spiritual home, to where the air is always a little clearer, the cares more distant, the pace of life – well, if not calmer (which the nightlife in the resort's very gay Yumbo Centre could never be described) – then certainly more assured and under control. Dennis and I had already had three holidays there so I was hardly a novice, and I booked myself into a very pleasant Brit gay complex called Vista Bonita, in the slightly more detached area of Sonnenland, overlooking the main resort of Playa del Inglés and Maspalomas. Using here as my base, I then proceeded to use the following three weeks 'fucking' Dennis out of my system, so to speak. Not to forget or to replace but, in some way that I never really analysed until many years later, to lay down new memories – fleeting if often fun – between the place that he had occupied in my life and where I now found myself. Or, as Mel commented dryly upon my return, it could just have been that I was a tart and one that even Dennis would have been far-pushed to equal in his single days.

There were, and I kept a good record, sixty-five 'encounters' across the twenty-one days although, to be fair, a few were the same guy and three were brothers (albeit not all at the same time). There were seven of these brothers, all Italian knife throwers from the Wild West Show at Sioux City, a tourist attraction in neighbouring San Agustin that survives to this day, with three of them gay – the youngest, the eldest and one in the middle, ranging from a barely legal 16 to 28 years. I should, perhaps, add that I did not seek out brothers number two and three but they had sought me, ostensibly, I later gathered, on the advice of the elder. What was more amazing was that I avoided even a single creepy crawly (*Pthirus pubis* or *Sarcoptes scabiei* to Latin scholars) let alone 'dose' in these three fine weeks but did find two friends whom I know to this day as well as one somewhat short-lived boyfriend.

Slowly – with setbacks – I started to move forward, progressing through a pattern of grieving, initially bumping along the bottom, then on a slow incline before falling back, then up on my feet again, ever finding myself just a little further forward. By the end of 1992, I was ready to start re-engaging with the world although, I must confess, I still remained a bit of a tart.

I first started exploring – this time with no sense of furtiveness – Portsmouth's gay scene, which while small was surprisingly well developed and diverse. With most of my gay friends inherited from Dennis and largely London-based, I soon started to make – for the very first time in my life – my own gay friends, from first principles, if you will. Through that, I also started to become engaged in local voluntary work – firstly with gay men's health and, subsequently, more specifically in the field of HIV and AIDS with a more regional and, eventually, London focus. I set up the Portsmouth Gay Men's Health Group, was invited to sit on other groups and boards and became a regular volunteer at 'London Lighthouse' where I worked on the 'Residential Unit', this being Europe's first HIV/AIDS centre and hospice. Eventually, all this would lead to my first paid position after the Navy, but of more relevance to me at that time was that it led to my discovering a support organisation for

LGBTQ veterans, called Rank Outsiders. It had been set up by Robert Ely and Elaine Chambers (whose own story can also be found in these pages) with the support of the LGBT lobbying organisation, Stonewall, the same year that I had left the Navy.

Early in 1993 I attended one of their first meetings, at Stonewall's first floor offices in Greycoat Place, Victoria, and was amazed to find a room packed full of people I had never met before but with one glaring thing in common: we had all lost our careers, either of our own volition or through being exposed and drummed out, from within Britain's Armed Forces.

This was a quite cathartic moment for me, and from that first evening, I not only embarked on many friendships that endure, strongly, to this day but it also – unknowingly to me at that moment – marked the start of something quite profound, which was to have repercussions felt across the world – certainly across the Atlantic – and that, while I may have forgone the prospect of command of my own warship, allowed me to play a key role in something that would make good for my lost career and my years before the mast.

While all that is a story picked up well by other companions and good friends amongst the contributors to this book, suffice to say that within a year I found myself taking over as the next Chair of Rank Outsiders. At the outset it was obvious that the best form of support we could provide to those who lived similar lives to ourselves (at a time in 1994 when it was still a criminal offence just to be gay in Britain's military, by which I mean with everything buttoned up and no clothes astray – with the possibility of detention at the previously mentioned Colchester and thereafter dismissed with their 'Services No Longer Required') was to remove the need for such support in the first case – and to campaign for the ban on gay men and women being able to serve openly in our Armed Forces to be lifted.

With Ed Hall and others, and Stonewall, the Armed Forces Legal Challenge Group was formed and, in due course, four from among many potential individuals were selected to have their cases taken, firstly to Judicial Review, then to the Court of Appeal (presided over by the Master of the Rolls) at the Royal Courts of Justice, and thence, skipping over the House of Lords, to the European Court of Human Rights. There, in September 1999, the Government of the United Kingdom was found in default and, in January 2000, I was able to sit in Strangers' Gallery alongside the Chief Executive of Stonewall and other friends and watch – without the need for any form of legislation – the ban being lifted by nothing more than a quiet and short statement from the Secretary of State for Defence, looking up, for a moment, at us in the Gallery.

It was then, merely for a instant, that I suddenly found myself back again in the scented pinewoods in the centre of Gran Canaria, near sunset – gazing out through the clear mountain air across to distant Tenerife, Dennis leaning against me and not a sound to be heard, not a bird's lifting song nor a cricket's chirp – just for one sparkling split second of eternity. 'There's still blossom in the trees,' he said. It was some while before I realised where I was, that people were shaking my shoulder and that, with a shiver, he had gone.

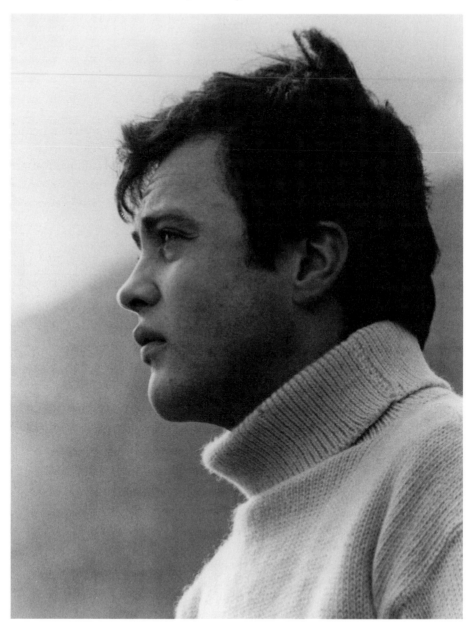

Northern Ireland, 1980.

Chapter 3
The Unsinkable …
Lieutenant Commander Craig Jones MBE
Royal Navy

My family link to the Armed Forces was tenuous; however, the service of an uncle as a radio operator shortly after the Second World War was enough to make us a naval family. My uncle had trained at what is now the Communications Warfare School at HMS Collingwood in 1953, an organisation that I was to command later in my career. And so, as a boy, I joined the 3rd Bingley Sea Scout Troop and five years later, found myself heading to Portsmouth University to undertake a degree in Economics, where I joined the University Royal Naval Reserve Unit.

In my first year at university I spent almost every weekend on the ship and my evenings at drill nights learning everything I could about the Royal Navy. After nine months, I applied for a reserved place as an officer and was invited to attend the Admiralty Interview Board. The AIB was a rigorous three-day assessment of a candidate's potential to be an officer; it was my one chance to realise my dream and I worked night and day to prepare. In the 1980s, competition to join the Royal Navy as an officer was tough and the odds were against me. By the time I arrived at the AIB in early May 1987, I knew every aircraft, ship and missile in the Fleet, their engines, their radars and their sonars. Over many weeks, I'd prepared for tests in general knowledge, numeracy, English and military, and I sailed through the

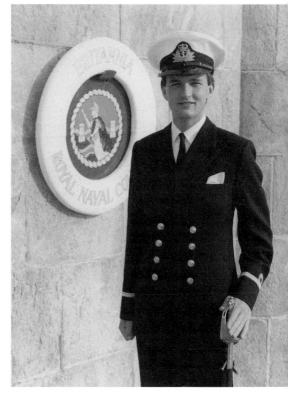

A uniform that I would need to grow into! Dartmouth, 1989.

first day, which focused upon these written hurdles. Day two involved leadership tasks, and the other candidates and I forded water tanks and imaginary streams and caverns with wood poles, rope, pulleys and barrels, taking it in turns to lead each evolution. My leadership task involved using ropes and planks to bridge a cavern to a platform. I was lucky and my task came late in the day, when our skills were quite polished. I sighed with relief when the last man reached the platform.

Our final day started with a one-to-one interview with a female lieutenant called the 'Personnel Selection Officer' (PSO). The Lieutenant invited me into the interview room. Unlike other rooms at the AIB, there were no pictures of ships or aircraft, and the furniture was distinctly unmilitary; two comfortable armchairs were positioned by a window, separated by a coffee table and a colourful rug. None of this eased me away from my guard. I knew what was coming. She beckoned me to one of the chairs and I sat down. She started with some questions about my family and school life. She asked if we were a close-knit family and enquired about my brother. She then moved on to ask about university life and about my course, enquiring about my social time, skilfully weaving into the conversation questions about drugs, alcohol and gambling. She seemed pleased with my answers. She then asked me about friends and enquired whether I had any gay friends. I have never been a good liar and it was a great relief to be able to say 'No', and I added that I'd never met anybody who was gay. This seemed a very agreeable answer and she moved her interview on to talk about my university course and my anticipated grade of degree. After forty-five minutes she seemed to have the answers she needed and brought the interview to an end. I was relieved to leave the room – was it possible that you could tell that somebody was gay just by looking at them? I had no idea. My board interview started with naval knowledge and the Commodore asked me to choose one of the ships depicted by photographs on the wall and tell him about it. I turned round and saw a picture of my own unit's patrol boat, HMS *Fencer* … Twenty minutes later, the Commodore interrupted to say that he'd heard quite enough about that patrol boat for one day, and so I won my place.

During the months of preparation for my final exams I often took time out to walk down to the dockyard and marvel at the warships that were moored sometimes two or three deep, many more alongside and still more in the creek beyond. It was then one of the largest military dockyards in the Western world and home to the majority of the Royal Navy's sixty-five or so frigates, destroyers and aircraft carriers. It was May 1989 and I was due to cross the threshold at Britannia Royal Navy College Dartmouth in just three months' time to commence my officer training, at a time when my young life's ambition was almost within reach. It was a prize I wanted for myself, but I also carried the hopes and aspirations of my family. With little doubt, my mother saw me in the future as the commander of a frigate, married to an admiral's daughter and living in a cottage in Hampshire with our two children, Charlotte and Henry, and a black Labrador. Life was to turn out differently.

On one of my journeys from the dockyard back to my student lodgings at Lorne Road, Southsea, that summer I passed a newsagent's and was drawn to the magazine shelf. I purchased a copy of the *Radio Times* and returned to my rooms. I was staying in a large Victorian house with a kindly couple, Jacob and June. They had a strong Christian faith and quite specific house rules. By then I had joined the Royal Navy Reserve and they seemed in some way reassured that this might define my values in some positive way. My room was on the top floor. I closed the door behind me and checked the handle to make sure it was shut, turning the old rim lock until the deadbolt clicked. I then sat on the bed and stared at the glossy magazine cover – and there he was staring back at me, resplendently dressed as Marius from *Les Misérables*: Michael Ball. I appreciate that in recent times the mention of Michael Ball might bring forth an image of Edna Turnblad from *Hairspray*, or even a villainous Sweeney Todd, but I can assure you that in the 1980s, he was in every respect the perfect Marius – and hot stuff. Quietly, while staring at the bottom of the door to my room for fear of being disturbed, I muttered under my breath, 'I'm gay'. Despite the fact that I was in an attic room at the end of a long corridor, I watched the bottom of the door for any shadow that might suggest I risked being overheard, and listened attentively before repeating the phrase 'I'm gay, I'm gay, I'm gay', a little louder each time. This was not the first time I had come to this conclusion. On reflection, my orientation had never been a grey area and I had had a range of gay crushes at school and university. However, today I was prepared to say to myself – audibly, undeniably, with certainty and forever – that I was gay. On that day I accepted that I was destined to be different, a matter about which I had no choice. From the time of my earliest realisation, I saw nothing wrong with me, but accepted that others would.

***

On 13 September 1989, a little before 4.00 pm, I drove through the gates of Britannia Royal Naval College in Dartmouth to begin the remarkable journey as a junior officer. We mustered on the parade ground in front of the magnificent towers and turrets created in 1905 by Sir Aston Webb. A feisty petty officer barked orders that few of us understood. My name was called in a list of cadets destined for 'Blake Division' and I gladly scuttled away to my accommodation. My group was escorted by a midshipman called Matthew Reed. He had joined the college from school at the age of 19 and would spend two years there. As a graduate my training was shorter, at just twelve months. Midshipman Reed had a shock of blond hair and an air of self-assurance and experience I had not encountered in somebody so young. If I had concerns about the conflict of my orientation with my career, the intensity of my first fourteen weeks of basic training certainly helped settle things down! From 0500 to midnight each day was crammed with activity: polishing, learning, running, jumping, more polishing and, occasionally,

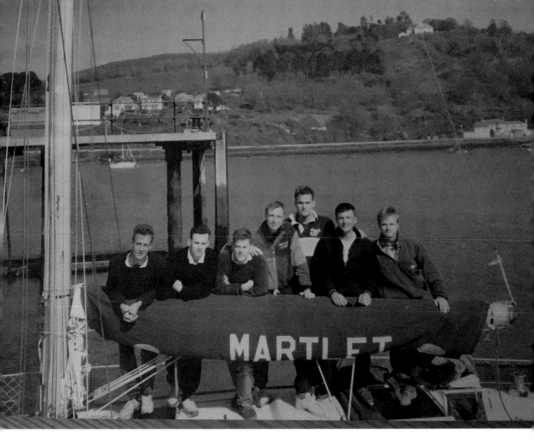

'The band of brothers' pictured on our divisional yacht, with Matthew Reed and I on the far right.

sleeping (but never for long enough). The only respite from the strenuous regime that prepares junior officers for service in the Fleet was representative sport. While at school I had raced sailing dinghies to notable success. Midshipman Reed was the captain of the college sailing team and he quickly found a place for me in the squad, and generally became my mentor. Thankfully, that involved weekends away from the college competing with the Royal Air Force and British Army, and I relished being freed from the exhausting activities at Britannia.

Matthew had bold confidence and was very well liked, and I was flattered to be included in his friendship group. He was fearless chasing a date and, much to everybody's amusement, he struck up a relationship with the daughter of the Dean of the college. In the first week of term he had a lucky escape one night climbing down the ivy from her bedroom in the grand house her family occupied on the edge of the parade ground. It was typical of Matthew: devil-may-care, assertive and always smiling. On reflection, I suspect his love interest with the Dean's daughter was not welcomed, and perhaps there was a sigh of relief as he left the girl behind when he completed training and joined the Fleet. Matthew was the first person in my life who epitomised the band of brothers that servicemen and women become when facing the challenges, adversity and hardships of service life. He 'looked out' for me during the greatest rigours of my training, and I benefitted from his brotherly kindness. Years later, when the wolves were at my door and chance brought our professional lives together, I took the greatest care to keep him clear of collateral damage.

The challenges of training were overcome and I was added to the list of cadets passing out at Lord High Admiral's Divisions on 5 April 1990, where the Princess Royal would take the royal salute. My parents planned to visit for the event with my brother and his girlfriend – but I was missing a belle for the summer ball that followed Lord High Admiral's Divisions. A few cadets would attend without escorts but I felt unreasonably conspicuous and wrote to an old school friend, Sarah. I booked a double room at a hotel in Dartmouth town. Quite frankly, this was a step too far in my wish to draw a smokescreen over the gaps in my life, but I got caught up in the moment. Whilst there may be folks out there who could 'carry off' finding a carrot in a bag of parsnips, I was not one of those, and finding myself in a room with Sarah after the ball would, at the very best, only end in disappointment for everybody! The two weeks leading up to Lord High Admiral's Divisions were peppered with anxiety. None of this was aided by being amidst a group of testosterone-fuelled cadets who had not seen their girlfriends for many weeks and eagerly anticipated all that the night would bring. My apprehension was in stark contrast, and each time I mentioned Sarah as my offering to the chatter about girlfriends, I couldn't help but feel that my expression of enthusiasm for the night was unconvincing. After a week of polishing my boots and sword, and the patent peak of my cap, the morning arrived. As I marched onto the parade ground, from the corner of my eye I spied my parents and Sarah. Whilst I was prepared to sign up to the principle of Nelson's 'band of brothers', I felt that he might need to take a rain check on the sentiment 'England expects that every man will do his duty', which was carved into the stone of the facade of the college.

The Princess Royal, in her role as Lord High Admiral, was driven onto the parade ground in a black Rolls-Royce. She stepped out to be greeted by the Commodore of BRNC, who escorted her to inspect us. She stopped and spoke to me, asking where I was to go next. Slightly unglamorously, I was joining a Fishery Protection Squadron vessel and she quipped that there was honour in protecting fish. As my career progressed, I would occasionally meet members of the Royal Family and I was always struck by the genuine interest they showed in our servicemen and women. Over the period of an hour, she presented swords and we offered a royal salute, lifting our swords skywards, crossing them on our chests and lowering the blade to the ground in deference. We then hooked up our scabbards and marched off the parade ground. After celebration drinks and a long lunch we all retired to prepare for the evening. I had agreed to collect Sarah from the hotel at 6.30 pm and began getting ready two hours before. I appreciate that, for many gay men, allowing two hours to get ready might seem not unreasonable. However, in this case, the passage of time had more to do with the challenge of the uniform.

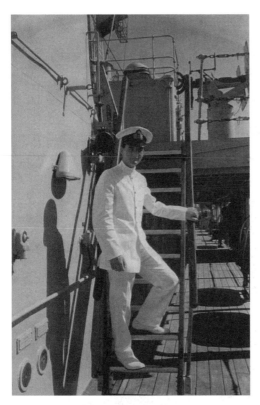

Hong Kong, and another complicated uniform! March 1990.

For a ball, an officer in the 1980s would wear No. 7 Mess Undress with white tie. In my twenty-year career I faced many great challenges, but few matched the complexity of donning this uniform. The shirt had a stiff front with gold screw-in studs, cufflinks and a detached stiff wing collar. In the list of military offences, buggering the Captain's dog was a lesser offence than wearing a pre-tied bow tie and, aside from being gay, I am also left-handed, which seemed to add to the challenge. There was then a white waistcoat with brass buttons, which needed cleaning and individually attaching (if you missed a dab of polish, it appeared as a green blob on the starched Marcella). The trousers were high-back cavalry style in heavy barathea, notably figure-hugging, and the ensemble was completed with a bolero jacket.

Any man who believed that gay men and women were not serving in the military needed to chat to the guy that designed the uniform. It remains an outfit fitting of the most impressive of state occasions, and this was the first time I had been allowed to wear it. The finishing touch was my Gieves & Hawkes mess boots, which remain in my wardrobe today, purchased at the outrageous cost of £200. In 1989, this fabulous ensemble – crafted by the best military tailors in the world – munched £1,200 of my uniform grant, but I begrudged not a penny, and it has stood the test of time. Even the most plain of young officers stood the chance of a conquest in this uniform … if they could get into the damn thing (or perhaps, more importantly, out of it!).

Even in these early days, imagining what it would be like to attend a ball or function with a boy on my arm seemed too scary to dwell on. I pushed it to the back of my mind and returned to the crocodile nearest my canoe – Sarah! But with unspoken consent, we happily parted company a little after midnight, with nothing said or expected.

***

After a few months with the Fishery Protection Squadron and my training now completed, I joined Type 22 Frigate HMS *Cornwall*, on station in Bermuda as our West Indies Guard Ship. It was a plum appointment and much envied by others on my course who had been assigned to ships involved in fishery protection, hydrographic survey or deploying to the Falkland Islands (where the greatest excitement was seeing the penguins). *Cornwall* was one of the largest ships in the Royal Navy, with 280 men and women and commanded by one of the most senior captains in the Fleet. For the majority of my service in this fine ship, she was commanded by Captain (later, Vice Admiral) 'Tom' Blackburn. Captain 'Tom' was a gentleman. A lifelong confidant of the Duke of Edinburgh who was later in his career to become the Master of the Royal Household.

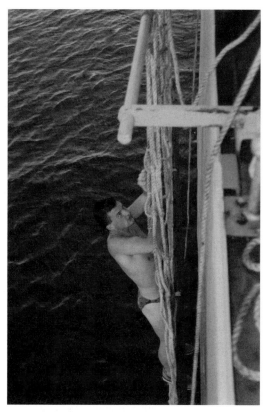

Hands to Bathe, HMS *Cornwall*, Caribbean, 1992.

I learned a great deal from him about subtlety in leadership and how much could be achieved by a calm, considered and measured approach.

To my surprise (on reflection), I took with me a large stuffed leopard named Tigger, gifted to me by my mother on my twenty-first birthday to replace an earlier version that was threadbare. Clearly the sentimentality of the stuffed toy overcame the potential simile to Brideshead's Aloysius. Tigger became a popular personality in HMS *Cornwall* and was kept on my bunk opposite the officers' pantry. The existence of Tigger seemed to be viewed as eccentric rather than 'a bit gay' and each morning on the bridge, Captain Tom would ask me how I was and how Tigger was finding the day. One morning, on returning to my cabin, Tigger had been swiped. I had the forenoon watch (0800–1200) on the bridge, so there was no time to search, and I fixed our position on the chart and took 'charge' of the ship from the officer handing over. The forenoon's activity involved calibrating our Lynx helicopter's gyro compass using the much larger gyros operated in the ship. Unusually, Captain Tom was in his chair on the bridge for what was quite a dull evolution. The helicopter thundered up alongside the bridge wing at the very

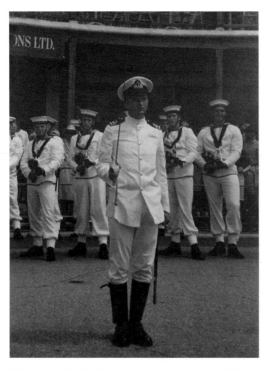

The Queen's birthday parade, Bermuda 2002 ... hoping nobody had rounds in the chamber!

close range needed to complete the calibration and I looked across from my position at the compass platform to signal to the pilot that we were ready to commence … and the furry paw of Tigger waved back from the pilot's seat. Captain Tom was sniggering with delight. A little over a week later, I was on the bridge driving us towards a fuel replenishment with a large fleet auxiliary tanker. It was a dangerous evolution for a frigate of over 5,000 tonnes and a tanker that was considerably larger. The ships were required to position themselves alongside each other while this was under way, and there was no room for mistakes. I was firmly focused on our distance from the tanker and Captain Tom reminded me to keep an eye out for other shipping.

Breaking my concentration, I tersely snapped back, 'Yes Sir', quickly scanned the horizon and returned my fixed gaze to the tanker. The replenishment completed, I handed the ship over to the afternoon watch and went down the ladders, past the Captain's cabin on my way to lunch. As I passed his door, Captain Tom beckoned me in and asked if he had irritated me on the bridge. The comment vexed me; he was one of the most senior, respected and admired officers in the Fleet and whether he might have irritated me seemed to have no relevance. I was a very junior lieutenant by then. The only answer I could offer was to assure him that this was not the case. I skipped lunch, went to my cabin and sat thinking for a while about the meaning of his comment, until 'the light turned on'. With great subtlety, Captain Tom had instructed me about how officers should treat each other. It was a clever admonishment by an officer who had far greater skills than fire and brimstone. Many years later, while a guest at Buckingham Palace, I was particularly pleased to cross paths with the then Vice Admiral Tom Blackburn, master of the Royal Household, after introducing him to my husband. His first words were, 'And how is our Tigger these days?'

After returning from the West Indies and a few weeks' rest, it was announced that we were to go to the northern Arabian Gulf. The Shatt al-Arab, a waterway that connected Baghdad to the open waters of the Gulf, had been clogged with ships and silted, and in the immediate aftermath of the first Gulf War, it needed clearing. There were concerns that as these vessels were floated and dragged into open waters, contraband, people or munitions could be smuggled, and boarding by boat was considered laborious and relied upon the goodwill of other regional protection forces. The Commander-in-Chief Fleet decided that a new approach was needed and HMS *Cornwall* was directed to 'stand up' a boarding team that would undertake these boardings by helicopter fast rope. Until then, helicopter fast rope (jumping out of helicopters on ropes) had been limited to Royal Marines, who undertook a more substantial course of training in combat warfare. I had some ground to catch up. After a week at

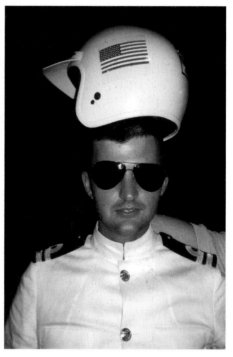

Letting off steam, West Indies, 2002.

the gunnery school at HMS Cambridge, taking apart and reassembling my 9mm browning pistol, my petty officer and I went to RAF Netheravon and completed a Helicopter Fast Rope Instructor course, joining a group of fifteen Royal Marines. Over a period of weeks we jumped out of a wide range of helicopters to practise our drills and, aside from a few minor ankle bruises and despite our blue uniforms, we seemed as competent as our dark green colleagues.

After an exciting few weeks, I returned to the ship on the Sunday night full of enthusiasm for sailing through Plymouth Sound the following morning at the start of our deployment. I stepped into the bar to find my fellow officers muttering in hushed tones. I grabbed a beer from the fridge and listened intently. Able Seaman Evans had left the ship accompanied by the Special Investigation Branch on Friday: apparently, he was gay. I was immediately struck by the compassion of my fellow officers. Nobody was gleeful at this turn of events, yet no one suggested it was unjustified; it was just necessary. I finished my beer and went back to my cabin, where Tigger was perched on my bed. It was fair to say that I was having the time of my life and this felt like a stark warning shot across my bows. It was the bluntest reminder of how quickly everything could be lost.

The following morning, I picked myself up and climbed the ladders to the bridge to don my headset to take HMS *Cornwall* through Plymouth Sound on the first leg of her journey to the Gulf – a fuelling stop in Gibraltar. On our way south, my petty officer and I selected our boarding team, which would include two Royal Marines who had been embarked for the deployment. We began their training as we dashed through the south-west approaches, starting with ropes suspended in the aircraft hangar and progressing to jumps from our Lynx helicopter onto the flight deck, bows and eventually onto the bridge wings. These were the first jumps we had made wearing bulletproof vests and with the extra weight, keeping control in descent was much more challenging. In the last twenty-five years, technology has improved the materials used to stop the passage of a bullet and the vests are now lighter and more compact, but in 1993, they were heavy and bulky. We completed our preparations by firing a few magazines from our pistols and rifles against a balloon target towed from the back of the ship. It burst on the first hit and the galley sent up a couple of their industrial scale baked bean tins, which were dropped from the quarterdeck to provide a shiny target in the clear blue waters of the Mediterranean.

After a swift transit of the Suez Canal, we sighted the Straits of Hormuz and the ship was brought to its highest state of readiness: 'Action Stations'. It was early

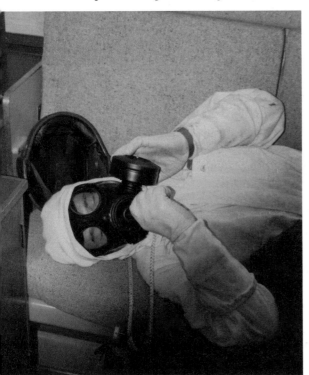

in 1993 and there remained a great deal of tension in the region. Little more than a year before, HMS *Gloucester*, under the Command of Captain 'Fighting Phil Wilcocks', had shot down a Silkworm missile bound for the battleship USS *Missouri* in the waters we passed through, and we remained at action stations for a few hours until the confined waters of the straits were behind us.

The Northern Sector of the Gulf was controlled by the USS *Nimitz*. At over 100,000 tonnes, this mammoth aircraft carrier was twenty times the size of a frigate. She commanded the water and airspace around her with notable firmness, and anything larger than a seagull risked being shot down for being off station. Soon after our arrival in theatre, *Nimitz* allocated us two vessels that were being

The Gulf, 1993. A restful moment in a gas mask, preparing for action stations.

towed clear of the Gulf to board. We were the first fast rope team to operate in the area, with US and allied nations launching boarding parties in a wide range of shabby motorboats. As our team prepared to board the Lynx, I felt some sense of occasion and had one of those 'the eyes of the nation' moments. Our Principal Warfare Officer, Lieutenant Commander Roly Woods, who had become a friend, shook my hand as I got into the helicopter, with the parting advice: 'Don't fall off the rope or shoot yourself in the foot.'

Our target vessels were a tug and tow. The towed vessel was the *Thalasini Mana*, which had been silted in the Shatt al-Arab for many months. Her tug was named *Dubai Moon*. We agreed to tackle the towed vessel first; she would be more complex to search and there was a greater chance of something untoward. After circling our target in the Lynx to observe the crew and the decks we made a steep decent to hover over the bridge wing. The bridge roof would have provided a flat and open site for

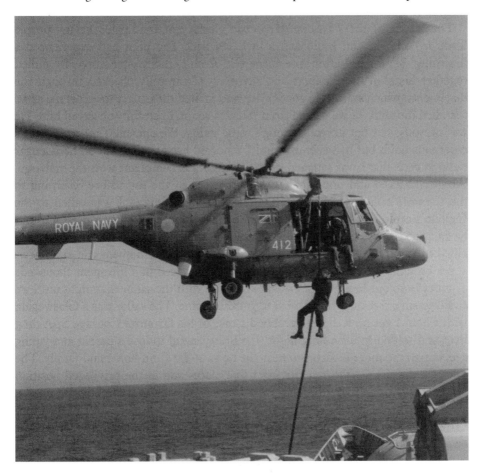

Departing the aircraft feet first, Northern Arabian Gulf, 2003, helicopter insertion boardings.

us to descend to; however, I was concerned about the radars mounted directly above and had no wish to get my team too close to their energy blasts. We dropped the ropes and left the aircraft for an uneventful 50-foot decent to the merchants' deck. The master had embarked a pilot who spoke perfect English. I deployed my team to the decks to take a look around, keeping my Royal Marine bodyguard close. Our sailors had the somewhat clumsy SA80 assault rifle, which was far from ideal when clambering around ships. The Royal Marines were carrying the Heckler & Koch MP5, a much sleeker weapon; reliable and with a shorter frame, it would have been my weapon of choice but as the only officer in the group, I got a Browning 9mm pistol. The Browning was designed in 1935 and was one of the simplest handguns in the world. My pistol came with a green canvas holster, which shrunk in contact with salt water to such an extent that it was virtually impossible to draw the weapon. I could not help but think that it might have been designed by the Army to be the weapon of choice for Royal Navy officers.

The master of the *Thalasini Mana* had clearly not anticipated having people 'drop in' on him and he looked a little startled. The pilot had experienced a 'boarding' before and after an exchange in Arabic, the master hurriedly pulled together his ship's log, papers and inventory. I carefully checked through the documents, which seemed in good order, and invited the master to escort me as we searched the ship. As we passed from room to room, I carefully observed him. He was nervous, but not nervous enough to be guilty. We opened *Thalasini Mana*'s cavernous hold, but it was empty and I reported back to the ship on my Cougar radio in code that I was satisfied that the vessel was compliant with the embargo. We disembarked and undertook a cursory check of the tug before returning to the *Cornwall*'s flight deck. Shortly after supper that night, I was called to the Captain's cabin. Captain Blackburn had a serious look, which surprised me, and he and our Executive Officer told me that the father of one of my men had been killed in an oil rig explosion in Mexico. It was a sombre moment and such news at sea brought back to us the vulnerability we all faced in a life spent thousands of miles from our loved ones. I was asked to sit with the sailor that night until we could steam a day early into Dubai to get him home. The sailor was a Glaswegian with whom I got on well, so I grabbed a case of his favourite Courage Sparkling Beer and settled in for a long night. It's pretty awful to lose a parent at a young age, but all the more difficult to hear the news so far from home and family. The role of a divisional officer at the front line places you in the privileged position of being able to make a difference, and I never took that duty lightly. He cried a great deal and we drank until he drifted in and out of sleep. Then I packed him a bag and as soon as the gangway went down in Dubai, he was whisked away in a taxi by the Naval Attaché.

***

After some weeks in the Gulf conducting our operations, we headed east for Singapore, where I was due to leave the ship, my tour of duty being completed. In my range of duties in HMS *Cornwall*, I was specifically responsible for the welfare of the ship's largest mess deck, which provided accommodation for fifty-seven men, defined by its location marking '3 Hotel Zulu' but known affectionately as 'The Zoo'. I was fortunate to be a popular officer with my teams and I spent a fair bit of time with them in the mess deck. There was a fine line between knowing when to arrive and when to leave. They were a lively bunch and many had served for more years than I had lived, but I had their best interests at heart and they took some pride in looking after their youthful 22-year-old officer. On special nights, such as returning up the Channel to our home port, I was never short of an invite – it was getting away that was more problematic! As we passed through the Malacca Straits, getting ever nearer to Singapore, I got the inevitable invitation to a leaving 'run ashore' at the famed Fire nightclub. By then I was a veteran of the 'run ashore' with the boys and had mastered the art of being in the right place at the right time and always finding the right moment to slip away. Once on a visit to Campbelltown, the leading seaman in charge of The Zoo had thrown me through the saloon doors of a pub to avoid me witnessing a fight between one of my sailors and a marine engineer from the ship. The next day at Captain's disciplinary table, I was able to represent him because I was not a witness to the altercation. It was good common sense and naval law at its finest.

We docked in Singapore and at 6.00 pm I appeared at the top of the hatch to The Zoo as directed. A tin of Courage Sparkling Beer was thrust in one hand and I was

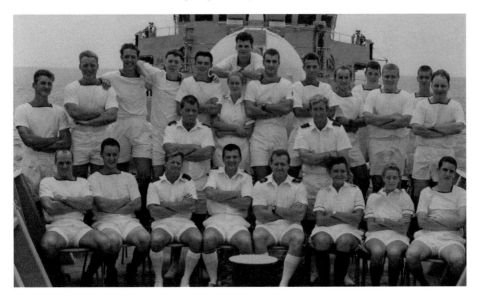

The Radar Division, HMS *Cornwall*, 1994, about a third of 'The Zoo'.

grabbed by my other hand and pulled through the hatch head first. All fifty-seven of my men were lined up for a photograph and the leading hand of the mess gave thanks for my time. It's not unusual to get a tankard or something akin at these occasions, and that was my expectation, but The Zoo had been imaginative. 'And tonight, Sir, you will be jetting off to Sembawang with Able Seaman Jarvis, where we have arranged two lovely ladies for you.' Rarely have I felt quite so horrified. Seemingly, it was a mess tradition to send the youngest member of the mess deck and their mess deck officer to a brothel – and these experienced tars knew just the place! More worryingly, Jarvis looked delighted with the idea. Although barely 18, he was a little over 6ft 3ins and had experience well beyond my boundaries. He really did seem to be very streetwise for such a young chap. He sidled up to me, rubbed his hands together and whispered collusively, 'We're gonna have a right old time, Sir, eh?' I took a long gasping swig of my CSB. It was certainly going to be a long night. 'Oh yes, can't wait!' I replied.

After a few more tins of CSB, the forty or so mess members who were not on duty stepped over the gangway in the direction of the nightclub. Fire was an eye-opener for an officer who had led a fairly sheltered life, but my sailors seemed to fit in very well indeed. Jarvis was enjoying the moment and holding court with a group of younger mess members who were exchanging ideas on techniques. I was with my leading hands, doing my level best to appear cool. Drinking seemed to help, so I kept going until Jarvis appeared in my shadow at a little after midnight. He had in

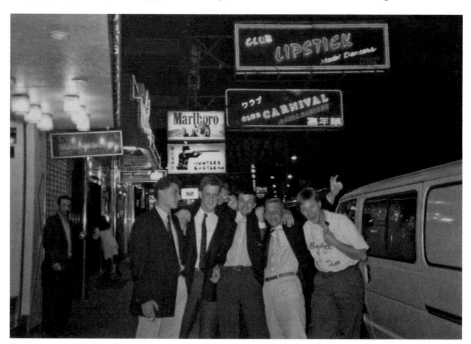

The 'Band of Brothers'.

his grasp a little over £90, which the mess had gathered up to send us on our way, and a few minutes later I found myself in a taxi en route to a brothel in Sembawang with Jarvis, who was in a state of noticeable enthusiasm. After the customary altercation with the taxi driver about the tip, we stumbled through the door of the 'Orchid Rooms' to be greeted by a 'manager' who looked like an extra from *Raging Bull*, as well as a lady who was a little over her teens and an older lady with rather thick make-up but a cheery face. Quick off his feet, Jarvis grabbed the hand of the younger lady and disappeared down a narrow corridor of rooms, and I heard a door shut behind them. At this point I theoretically had two options. I could have run, but I was in a tricky area of Sembawang, and Jarvis, with his stature and streetwise manner, was my safe ticket home. The older lady beckoned me with her painted finger to follow her, saying, 'I'm Mae – what about you?' I mumbled 'I may not' under my breath and followed her. There seemed little choice.

The room was dimly lit and had an air of Yardley about it. There was a bed with a candlewick bedspread and a shower in the corner, which would not have passed muster for Captain's rounds, and an equally grubby looking fridge. ... And then I took an enormous risk. I had never 'come out' to anybody, but there was a kindness in her eyes and I really couldn't see an alternative, so I sat down by her side and, with a conspiratorial tone, I told her I was gay and needed to make sure that Jarvis was none the wiser. She seemed quite pleased and explained that all that discretion would be expensive. I gave her the £40 that Jarvis had left me with. Given that her duties would be limited, it seemed very fair to me, but she looked a little disappointed, so I slipped her another £40, which lightened the mood. 'Go water hair look wet, go shower, shower, shower, shower,' she said emphatically. With an eye on my wallet, I followed the instruction, then dried off and got dressed again. She opened the fridge and grabbed two Tiger beers and we sat on the bed and cracked them open. Every five minutes she got up and opened a wooden flap on the wall, through which she could see into the room next door, where Jarvis was no doubt quite busy. After three or four checks, she said, 'Hey sailor, he's leaving – you wait another five few minutes. Officer should last longer!' With my time up I moved towards the door and the cheery lady asked for another £20. 'What for?' I asked. She pointed at the Tiger beer cans. She had a point and this seemed a poor time to haggle. I opened the door and saw Jarvis at the end of the corridor in a James Dean pose leaning against a door frame, bare-chested with his T-shirt nonchalantly over his shoulder and a cigarette drooping from his mouth. As I walked towards him, Mae shouted after me, 'You Lieutenant got huge cock, very hard, you come again I give you big discount.' There was honour in her trade. Jarvis looked a little less cocksure by the time I got to him.

We jumped in a cab and returned to the ship. For my remaining forty-eight hours in HMS *Cornwall* I was a legend, and I basked in the sun.

***

My appointment in HMS *Cornwall* had been a great success and my skills at ship driving and leading had been carefully noted in my annual reports. In consequence there was a range of roles on offer, but the one that caught my eye was Executive Officer of a Northern Ireland patrol boat. I had thrived in the operational environment of the Gulf and had military skills in boarding operations and weapon craft that were seldom achieved by young officers employed in warships. Northern Ireland was experiencing a bloody period in its history and I relished the opportunity to be involved in an operational environment where I could add value. It seemed the perfect fit and I gladly accepted an appointment to HMS *Itchen*.

Itchen was a River class minesweeper that had been substantially modified to take a Royal Marines boat group. In preparation, I undertook more weapons and comprehensive threat training, to improve my awareness of the mortars being used by the IRA. There were also grave concerns about the use of sniper rifles in the border areas and the Royal Navy were considered significantly at threat. *Itchen* was a command platform for Operation Interknit, which was the patrol of the eastern border on Carlingford Lough and Operation Grenada, which was the patrol north from Carlingford around the coastline to Lough Foyle and Londonderry. Teams of Royal Marines from HMS *Itchen* and her sister ships boarded ferries from Warren Point and Belfast bound for the UK to check for known personalities, bombs, guns and contraband. We also mounted amphibious vehicle checkpoints, using the boat group to mount the beaches and move onto the road. Army units on the roads were carefully monitored and 'dicked' (reported on) by both the Republican and Protestant terrorists, and these operations mounted from the sea often caught sympathisers off guard. There was also the opportunity to board fishing vessels along the coastline in the hope that we might be passed some intelligence – and if we didn't get intelligence from the fishermen, a lobster or a bit of halibut was always welcome. My greatest challenge was potcheen and sloe gin, used by many of the fishermen to stave off the cold winter in the Irish Sea. Alcohol and guns are a poor mix, but I always felt ungrateful at not sharing a dram with the fishermen on my patch. Whatever their faith or politics, most of those I met simply wanted to continue their lives without the chaos of this pointless and increasingly bloody war.

My team for boarding operations depended on the size of the vessel. For a small fisherman, the Royal Marines would drop off our military policeman and me, and possibly a sniffer dog if we had one embarked. Our military policeman was Regulating Petty Officer Tatcher. We got on very well, but like so many of his fellow rozzers, he didn't have a strong understanding of the need for discretion, and in the presence of a crime, was like a dog with a bone. He was also a stickler for rules, something that made me nervous in front-line operations. There were times when initiative was needed, rather than rigidity. Tatcher tended to board fishing boats and pleasure craft with me. If there was a larger vessel or a ferry, we would send two bricks of Royal Marines (2 x 4) plus me and a bodyguard. In

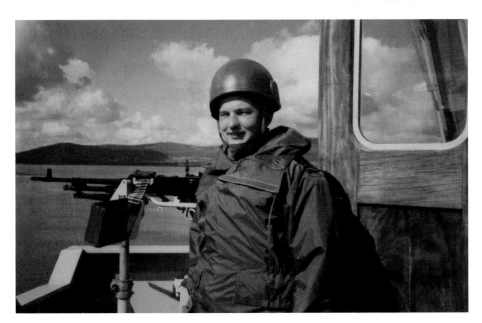

Entering Carlingford Lough, 1994, weighed down by body armour!

Northern Ireland there was a greater necessity to my having a bodyguard, because the most belligerent of locals knew what an officer's beret badge looked like. That made me the target of quite a few punches and I was always pleased when my Royal Marine got a block in the middle.

I settled into the routine very well and in my first year worked longer days than at any time in my career. It was a tough time in Northern Ireland, during which there were many civilian and military deaths that gave our teams an acute sense of the importance of their work. We spent much of our time guarding the border on Carlingford Lough, but would occasionally trip up the coast to Kilkeel or Bangor for a change of scene and the possibility of some fresh fish. Once every couple of months, I disembarked the ship for forty-eight hours for intelligence briefings in Belfast with the RUC, Army Intelligence officers and some unshaven but clearly military individuals whose background was never discussed, but over the years it became clear that they were members of the Special Reconnaissance Unit, or 14th Intelligence Unit, as it was also known. These highly skilled and courageous undercover operatives provided background intelligence for Special Forces operations in Northern Ireland. Out and about daily on our 'beat', Tatcher and I were well positioned to provide information about the movements of people in the border regions, but in consequence, our faces were well known and we were at higher risk of a targeted attack.

In December 1993, our sister ship, HMS *Cygnet*, had come under fire from an IRA sniper using a 0.5 inch Barrett lite sniper rifle. This deadly long-range

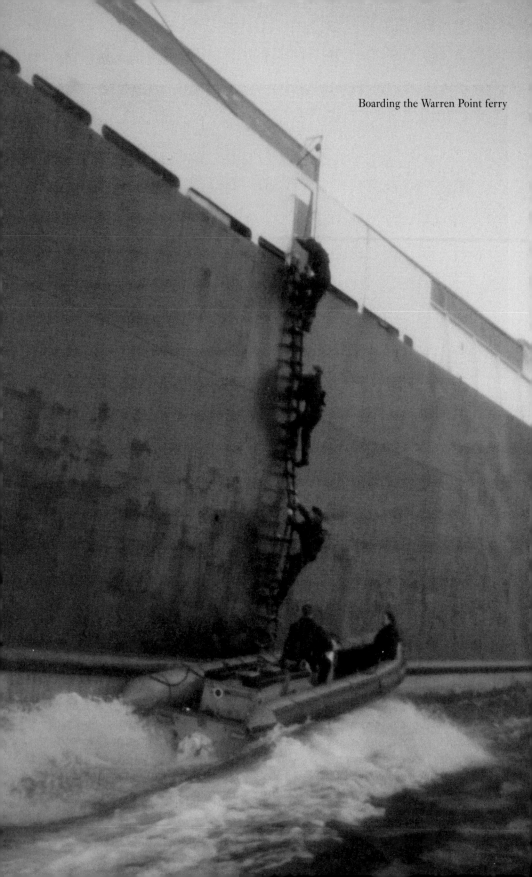

Boarding the Warren Point ferry

weapon discharged the bullet with huge kinetic energy and it could pass straight through the flak jackets in use at the time. It caused many deaths in Northern Ireland during my time there and was a silent and stealthy killer. The crew of *Cygnet* had dodged the bullet because the IRA had misjudged the range of the vessel and the bullets fell short.

We took as much care with our personal security as we sensibly could, never travelling in uniform without a 9mm pistol in a holster, or strapped to our chest when in civilian clothing. Although a flagrant breach of the rules, my pistol was permanently loaded and hung on my cabin door, ready to go. By the book, it should have been loaded and unloaded for each operation, but sometimes we got little notice of where the bad boys were on our beat, and every second counted. We were often exhausted, and each load and unload while mentally and physically shattered increased the chances of accidentally putting a round in the chamber – an almost daily event somewhere in Northern Ireland.

Getting me to Belfast for my monthly briefings was an uncomfortable and dangerous process called a 'green move'. Our Royal Marine troop mounted the beach in the rigid raiders in a prearranged position on the northern coastline of Carlingford Lough, where we would meet three Snatch Land Rovers loaded with heavily armed soldiers. With the Royal Marines on the beach and the soldiers in the Snatch vehicles ready to provide covering fire, I would then walk across the no

Maritime patrol off Kilkeel.

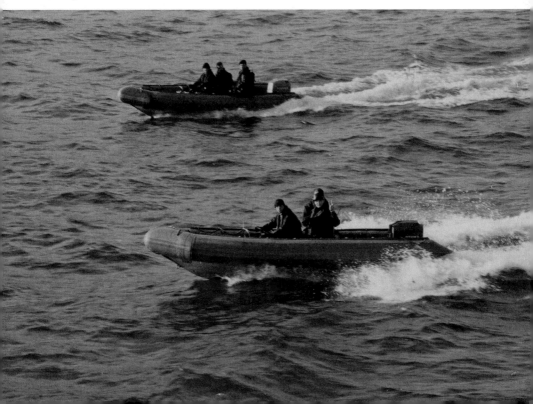

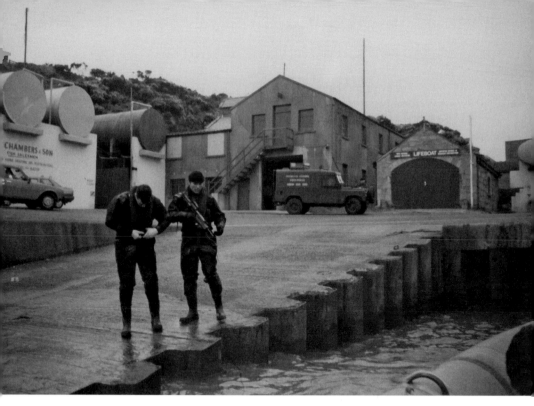

Green Move, Kilkeel, 1994.

man's land of the beach to meet them. Although only 100 yards, those walks were some of the longest of my life.

In November 1994, I completed my last green move of the year and arrived in Belfast at the Intelligence Centre for briefings. It had been a grim few months and the discussions that would eventually lead to the Good Friday Agreement had brought more instability than peace. The briefing painted a picture of very high levels of volatility and indiscipline in both Protestant and Republican paramilitary organisations, and it seemed that we were now increasingly at risk from both sides of this bloody war. In the margins of the briefings, there was a chance to talk to my family and restock on little luxuries to take back to *Itchen*. I was conscious that this would be my last chance before Christmas to do some shopping, so I put on some civilian clothing, strapped a 9mm pistol onto my right shoulder and donned my Harris Tweed jacket. I tended to wear a jacket rather than a coat because it would be easier to draw the weapon if needed. I'd booked a car to drop me off and collect me an hour later. I was rarely on the streets in civilian clothing in Belfast and whenever possible, I left my errands until my return to the mainland. Although we took great care to avoid advance planning of trips into the city, there was always the chance of a vehicle or driver or me being recognised, and the IRA had proven remarkably proficient at responding to opportunity targets. The driver dropped me on the high street, outside Dunnes department store, and I quickly left the car and slipped through the door into the crowd. The store was already showing signs of preparations for Christmas and as I walked through the cosmetics section, there were piles of box sets. Dressed in my jacket I was a target for the loitering assistants with their tester bottles. I walked purposefully and grabbed the lift up to the first floor in search of a new shirt. It was while meandering through the menswear section that I first noticed that I was being monitored. He was tall, perhaps over 6ft and wearing a denim jacket, checked shirt and jeans. I avoided looking directly at him but glanced as nonchalantly as I could to see if it was possible that he might have a weapon. He was clearly watching my every move and didn't seem to care that I might have noticed. I made mental notes so I could describe him later to the Intelligence team. He was young, perhaps no more than 20, of athletic build. He had one earring, and it was forefront in my mind from the morning's briefing that there were fresh faces in the ranks of the IRA and loyalist paramilitaries as the most belligerent dissidents looked for a new generation of operatives to replace an old guard that had lost much of its appetite for the armed struggle. I continued to observe him carefully, moving behind a Christmas display and towards the tills to see if he followed me, which he did, getting closer and closer. I scanned the shop for accomplices but could not see anybody else with whom he might be working, and the first floor of a department store seemed an unlikely place for him to move in. Then he looked straight at me and walked towards me. I lightly held the corner of my jacket to locate my pistol and make sure it was not visible, when he walked right up to me and said, 'So what are you doing then?' in a soft brogue. 'I'm Army,' I growled. 'I know,' he said with a cheeky smile. 'That's what all the cute hot Army officers wear.' I recoiled in shock: this was not the risk I was expecting and I was dumbstruck. The best I could offer was a stuttered 'What?' Many soldiers had fallen foul of 'honey pot' abductions, but I'd never heard of a gay version of that. Could it be possible? Either way, it was a bad idea to stick around and find out. I had to get away. I pushed past him and hastily went down the stairs onto the street. As I neared the steps to the ground floor, I heard an exaggerated 'Excuse me' – but I didn't look back. I dashed along the high street and found a café from which I could see my pickup place and waited an agonising twenty minutes until the blue MG metro arrived with my driver. I got in quickly and he drove off. 'No shopping then, Sir?' 'No, nothing that I really fancied,' I lied.

In the first few months of 1994, we received a closely guarded classified message to inform us that the Chief of the Defence Staff, General Sir Peter Inge, would visit the ship on Carlingford Lough. The plan was to winch him down using a Wessex aircraft. This was all achievable, but not something we practised day to day, particularly with an officer well into his sixties, so it needed some preparation. The General would tour the ship and have lunch in the wardroom. I spoke to our leading cook and he suggested that the General might like a bit of lobster, so we weighed anchor and sailed north towards Bangor to make friends in the fishing community! Tatcher and I donned our black drysuits, grabbed our pistols and

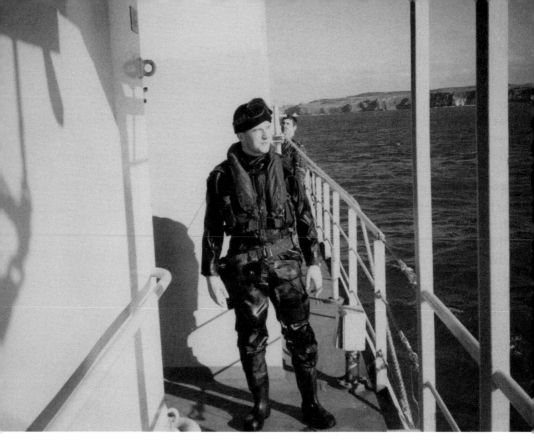

Tooled up and ready to go, Bangor.

scoured the horizon for a potter. About 3 miles south of Bangor, we spotted a large two-deck potter and closed in for the kill. As we approached, it was apparent that there was nobody on deck. The boat had a Bangor registration plate and we were able to make checks on its ownership to a sufficient level of reassurance to form the view that the crew were down below having supper (hopefully not the lobster we hoped to grab for the General!). Tatcher and I approached the potter's low decks and I jumped over, helping my fellow boarder make his leap. It was all too quiet. I unclipped the webbing strap keeping my gun in place and slipped my hand over the pistol grip. Keeping as much cover as possible, I stuck my head through the tight hatch to the accommodation deck below. To my shock, there he was, the boy from Dunnes, on a mattress in the arms of another young lad on the deck of the main cabin. They heard my feet on the ladder and were now hurriedly grabbing for their clothes. The boy from Dunnes looked at me in disbelief. In 1994, the age of consent in the UK was 21 and the younger of the two was certainly a few years short of that. My zealous military police colleague would have loved to get his policeman's notebook out so he could retell this tale in the senior rates' mess. I stood in the middle of the hatch blocking Tatcher's view. 'Everything all right down there?' he said. 'Yes,' I replied, adding that the crew were just resting. I caught the eye of the guy from Dunnes and he raised a grateful eyebrow. When I stepped out of the hatch, Tatcher looked at me quizzically, so to distract him I instructed him to search the cockpit before they got there. The bloodhound in him was sated by the possibility of a find, and he quickly set to task, opening drawers and cupboards. Not more than a minute later, the two young men appeared in the cockpit, in a state of mild undress and with tousled hair. Before they could speak, I said they must have had a busy day's fishing and been tired. With discernible relief, they nodded. Tatcher was every bit the detective and asked why they had no fish. The older of the two boys neatly replied that they were pulling the pots for repairs. It was unconvincing to me, but Tatcher seemed to let it go. We stayed a few minutes more and then left them to their day. Back on board the *Itchen*, Tatcher and I went to the wardroom to write our boarding reports for the day and behind the closed door he asked me directly if they were 'shagging'. I lied and sniggered as casually as I could, but he seemed unconvinced. In my remaining months on board I formed a view that Tatcher knew I'd covered something up and there was an air of distrust. He was a good man, loyal to his service and true to the regulations he was there to uphold, but if I slipped up, he would do nothing less than his duty as he saw it.

The boarding incident bothered me for some weeks afterwards. I was pleased that the boys had slipped away on their boat, perhaps shaken but otherwise safe. But for me, I had churned up the water around a void in my life. The pace of operations in HMS *Cornwall* and then in HMS *Itchen* had left little time for anything other than work, but I was 25, and in the weeks that followed I came to accept that I was hiding from the life I was destined to lead and that taking no risk in life would lead to a lonely outcome. Those two young men seemed to have the courage to be themselves, which I could not have dreamed of at their age. Courage comes in many forms and despite my beret, body armour and pistol, I felt like a coward. For over three years, I had immersed myself in some of the most high intensity military operations of the 1990s, but was I running to where my help was needed or running away from matters I could not face? The question left me shamefaced and I resolved to find as much honesty as my complicated life would allow.

After Christmas leave and a docking period, we sailed back into Belfast Lough for my last few months of my long tour of duty. There had been an unprecedented number of attacks early in the new year, and security was very tight. I had been due to go home to Yorkshire for my first weekend off in early February. However, I was instructed to vary my travel plans and I booked a flight to Exeter to visit Roly Woods, my old friend from HMS *Cornwall*. Roly lived in a large guesthouse, which he owned with his mother, Alice. They were assisted by a lodger called Peter, who was 24, tall and strikingly handsome. That night, after an evening out in Exeter at a bar that to me seemed extremely Bohemian, I had a little too much Dutch courage and 'came out' to Roly, and he confirmed that Peter was in fact a little more than a lodger! And so I started my first gay friendship. Now I really did have something to hide.

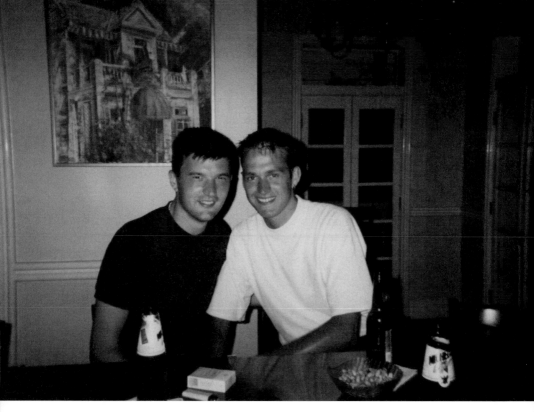

Adam and I escaping for our first holiday together - Key West, 1995. The world was suddenly in brilliant technicolour and I had never been happier. Whatever the future brought, we would face it together.

There was a lot to take in and I couldn't help but feel an unnerving ground rush. The following morning, we stepped out into a new world and sauntered along the road to the Exeter Arts Centre coffee shop, which was popular with the 'boys' on a Saturday lunchtime. As I walked through the door, amidst an exited and jolly crowd of young men, I spotted Adam on the far side of the room in a denim shirt and white T-shirt; he had a look of the *Footloose* about him. He was tall, neither blond nor dark, and quite a few years younger than me. I was transfixed and knew instantly that my life was about to become a great deal more complicated. We went on our first holiday together two weeks later over Easter leave … and the rest is our history!

***

In the summer of 1995, I left Northern Ireland for a long period of well-earned leave and to prepare myself to be the navigator of the frigate HMS *Sheffield*. Adam, then 19, had gone back to college to improve his grades and we spent the summer learning simultaneous equations and quadratics! It was a wonderful time in my life and my smile beamed from ear to ear. HMS *Sheffield* was a fine ship with over 200 crew, and I was excited by the new appointment. I completed the

Frigate Navigator's Course in the autumn and joined straight after Christmas. My career was soaring, and I had found the missing part of my life and was walking on clouds. It would be a very long fall from grace.

In the second week of January, Adam's father (who was separated from his mother) very suddenly dropped dead. It's the type of turn of events that the military manage in their stride every day, affording servicemen and women compassionate leave to support them to resolve issues at home such that they can continue their service duties with necessary reassurance. That system was not available to me and as HMS *Sheffield* sailed from Plymouth, I felt as though I had abandoned the love of my life. Still in shock, Adam was suggesting taking a break from his studies. So early in his task of crafting a new pathway for his life, I was determined that that should not happen. The best way I can describe the twenty-four hours that followed would be to say that it was, for this young lieutenant, 'all a bit much'. In frigates, navigators are in short supply. There were no others on board who could jump into the role for anything other than the short term; all other officers had their own roles. It was apparent that I was unfit to continue and a helicopter was swiftly raised to bring the Squadron Captain and a relief navigator on board and get me to hospital, where I remained for twenty-eight hours under sedation.

An hour's discussion with a surgeon captain psychiatrist established that I was not suicidal and I was sent on long leave. In my hospital bed I'd spent my time making lists in my head of things I needed to do to resolve the challenges at home. I was far from suicidal; I was going to be busy sorting things out and getting back to work. Nevertheless, this was a time of great sadness. I had shot a torpedo into my career that would take years to patch up.

When matters at home had been resolved as best they could, Adam and I decided a holiday was needed. In February, sunshine and warmth is in short supply in the northern hemisphere so we boarded a plane to The Gambia. There was a bit of civil unrest going on there, but it wasn't Belfast! On our second morning, I was sat at the bar reflecting on a chaotic period in life, when a man of a similar age, who I had seen with his boyfriend, sat on the stool next to me and said, 'You look bloody miserable.' In recent weeks I had come perilously close to losing a service career that mattered a great deal to me and exposure to the risk had curiously taken the edge off my nerves amidst my newly found gay bretheren. I flicked open my wallet on the bar, showed him my military ID card and said, 'That's because I've got one of those [pointing at the ID card] and one of those [pointing at Adam].' Sergeant Darren Ford, Royal Military Police, flicked open his wallet and revealed his Military Police warrant card, then pointed at his boyfriend. I hadn't considered that anybody else could be worse off! With great sadness, I discovered eighteen months later that his boyfriend outed him to the Royal Military Police and Darren was required to resign. He was a remarkable police sergeant and the Army lost one of its best.

My penance for leaving HMS *Sheffield* was to be sent as the third navigator of an aircraft carrier (when in fact an aircraft carrier only has two navigators!). It was a made-up job, sharpening pencils on the bridge, but it was where my complicated life had led me and I was determined to be the best pencil sharpener in the Fleet, if that was what was needed. HMS *Illustrious* was commanded by Admiral Sir Jonathan Band, a good man with fondness for cigars and rugby. He was a charismatic and well-respected leader. Sadly, I would never be an officer he could fathom, but that was not entirely his fault. I suspect he was mystified at my departure from *Sheffield* and very keen that I should return to navigate a frigate or destroyer to 'finish the job'. In my confidential report, Captain Band described me as 'intense and private with a reserved personality and worried manner'. He also noted – as was the reporting tradition at the time – that I was single. Much as the report burned in my mind like a fire, it was the man I had become – it was the damage done. Little more than twelve months earlier, my final confidential report on leaving Northern Ireland had described me having 'personal qualities beyond reproach, honest, loyal and courageous'. It continued that I was 'confident in all I did, a generous, charming host with a sharp wit', recommending me for early promotion and to command a small ship.

There were no questions that Captain Band could have been asked that would have helped me or I could have answered honestly. I faced this alone. Perhaps more than anything, this painful epoch laid the foundation of my bold and challenging reaction to the poor treatment of LGBTQ servicemen and women from the moment I could stand our corner. They had suffered enough.

And then the turn of fate rounded the right corner. As part of my penance I was from time to time given additional tasking. One of these tasks was to organise the visit of Captain Roy Clare CBE, who was to be the new commanding officer of our sister ship, HMS *Invincible*. It wasn't a task I relished, but it needed to be done, and done well. I rolled up my sleeves and got on with it, meeting Captain Clare on the gangway with a programme that filled every minute and ran like clockwork. He was briefed by our weapons and marine engineers, our aircrew, our bridge and operations room teams, and he had dinners and lunches in each of our messes and spent time with Captain Band. As I bade him farewell on the gangway at the end of his visit, he asked me what would be next in my career. It was a question that was difficult to answer and I stumbled on my words, finally managing to tell him that HMS *Invincible* needed a deputy navigator. He smiled, nodded and agreed to make some calls. A few weeks later, I walked across the dockyard for a new ship and a new start. I have no knowledge of what Captain Clare knew about my 'difficult year', but as I joined HMS *Invincible*, I remember feeling safe.

***

It was late 1997, and the furore of the debate about 'gays in the military' was a national news story that developed week by week. Admiral Sir Jock Slater, then First Sea Lord, printed an open letter in a national newspaper defending his position that the exclusion should continue. He was well supported by British Army and Royal Air Force service chiefs and the case seemed won for now. His successor as First Sea Lord, Admiral Sir Nigel Essenhigh, was widely rumoured to have threatened to resign if the prohibition was lifted. One lunchtime, I was sat in the wardroom on board discussing the situation with a group of young lieutenants and I heard myself say that I simply hoped we would 'never have to serve with those kinds'. Shortly afterwards, I left and went to my cabin. I slid the door closed and, not for the first time, sat at my desk with my head in my hands. It was a shocking moment of Judas and I was thoroughly ashamed of myself. I vowed it would never happen again; no matter what the risk, I would never deny who I was. An economy of the truth might be acceptable, but a lie was not. My first moment of being tested was to come very soon afterwards.

I got on with Captain Clare very well. He had a reputation for nurturing the careers of young officers and was an inspiring leader. Specifically, when he entertained senior officers in his dining cabin, he always shared the occasion with one or two more junior officers and I was delighted to have received an invitation card to a lunch where he would host the commodores of the main Royal Navy shore bases in Portsmouth (HMS Sultan, HMS Nelson, HMS Collingwood and HMS Excellent). The lunch was a jovial affair, bringing together a group of contemporaries who knew each other from many previous ships and roles. It went well and we worked our way through three courses of delicious food prepared in the Captain's private galley. As the cheese and biscuits were served, the discussion turned to 'gays in the military'. This was not altogether unusual; despite the unease of some, the most senior officers were generally keen to defend their position. At the lunch, the discussion was strong and loud and passionate. Captain Clare I thought would be the last to speak, and I doubted my opinion would have any importance; in fact, I expected to be overlooked. Captain Clare thought otherwise, and like a stray missile, the question came: 'And so, Craig, what does a younger officer think of gay men and women serving?' I had made my promise and carefully considered and accepted the risks. I understood my duty; there were no options for me. With a stony face and a seriousness and gravity that was to become a hallmark of my most difficult discussions, I reminded the commodores that they had spent fifteen minutes discussing slow progress in the procurement pipeline for new aircraft carriers to replace the ageing *Invincible* and *Illustrious* and well over half an hour discussing 'gays in the military'. I continued that if the First Sea Lord devoted more of his precious time petitioning for new carriers and less time trying to stop gay men and women from serving (which they were doing anyway) then perhaps we might all do better. There was a stony silence and tangible discomfort. It was not the response expected. Admiral Clare threw me a life ring. 'You're quite right, Craig. We sound like dinosaurs and it will be good leadership to see the ban lifted.'

After the dinner I retired to my cabin, proud to have found my voice but feeling vulnerable from the experience. The next day, during 'stand easy' (morning coffee, in Navy parlance), the main broadcast sounded and I was called to the Captain's cabin. I dashed up the ladders (there's an anticipated expediency to such orders barked on the main broadcast). After knocking with appropriate firmness, I put my head around the curtain on his door. He beckoned me in and pointed to an editorial at the foot of *The Times*: the headline read 'Writing on the Wall for Gay Ban'. 'They seem to agree with us,' retorted Admiral Clare. He handed me the paper and said, 'Take it.' (Because of the shortage of up-to-date newspapers at sea, there is a tradition of them being passed around.) I thanked him and left without further comment. After the ban was lifted I wrote to Admiral Clare to ask if he had seen beneath my cloak. With great warmth he remarked that he had not, but knew without a shadow of doubt that the continued exclusion of gay servicemen and women was wrong.

Through the bleak years, I was constantly aware that it would be all too easy for Adam to take a view that my much beloved Royal Navy was in some way an unwelcoming organisation or indeed one that did not place great importance on the role of our families. The reality is that the service greatly values the support that our families offer. He needed to understand the service and as he went to Sussex University in 1997, I very strongly encouraged him to join the University Royal Naval Unit, reflecting back on my time in HMS *Fencer*. I coached him for his interview and polished his shoes the night before. By then he knew far more about the service than any ordinary student and within weeks, he had a midshipman's uniform and an ID card. In a very positive environment he developed his own love for the service and experienced short summer and Easter deployments in his unit's patrol boat. It was not an aircraft carrier, but it was grey and flew a white ensign, and that seemed to be enough. He learned to coil ropes, put lines of pencil on charts, and which way to pass the port and Madeira. It was a terrific experience until he came home one day after 'drill night' and told me his new commanding officer had joined. 'Fantastic,' I said, 'what's his name?' 'Matthew Reed' was the answer. I hadn't seen Matthew for a few years. Our deployments had taken us to different ships in different parts of the world, but I considered him a close friend and, like all my fellow officers, did not wish him to be burdened by keeping my secret. Adam and I agreed that we would carry on provided that I had no contact with Matthew. Then, one evening, Matthew called me from Brighton Marina to say that he was bringing his little ship in for the night and would love to come round for a 'catch-up'. As I put the phone down, Adam and I looked around the room, our eyes falling on a Shirley Bassey tour poster – we needed to urgently 'de-gay' the flat. In a scene reminiscent of *The Birdcage*, we dashed around for an hour removing all traces of style, trying to create a 'bachelor pad'. After his visit that evening, Adam resigned from the URNU. He'd had a great time, but it was our problem and not a burden to be shared. Adam's time in the URNU was to have been of great importance, though. When the time came, Adam walked across the brows of ships and into wardrooms and messes with the confidence, bearing and courage of conviction of a member of the Officer Corps.

My appointment to *Invincible* went well and Admiral Clare recommended me for staff training and the prestigious Principal Warfare Officer's Course. The course was the foundation for becoming a senior officer in my branch and I was delighted. However, it would give me access to closely guarded military secrets and it was necessary that I be security cleared to routinely see information marked 'Top Secret' or that was so secret it had unique code words with access nominated individually by name and rank. Security clearance at that level made it likely that I would be exposed. For many years, Adam and I had shared bank accounts, mortgages and a home. Those ordinary connections of life were backed up by comprehensive records, to which military vetting officers had access.

And so, with mixed feelings, I bade farewell to Admiral Clare and walked down the gangway of HMS *Invincible* for the last time and moved on to the Military Staff College at Bracknell. If my career was to be curtailed by simple honesty, was it really all to be ended in Bracknell? It seemed an unlikely place for my last stand. And so the letter came in the post. I was to be interviewed by a retired colonel from the Defence Vetting Agency. It was May 1999, and my colleagues were thoroughly absorbed in the European Cup Finals and thankfully sufficiently distracted to not notice my personal disquiet as I counted the days to my interview and reminded myself that I would never again deny who I was. Although it was then less than 100 days from the European Court Ruling, my career would nevertheless end within twenty-four hours of disclosure. I met the Colonel in an interview room in a small military police unit at Bracknell. There were two chairs and a table. We shook hands. He was an older officer, dressed in tweeds, who looked at me over his half-moon glasses and invited me to sit down. Over the hour that followed, we discussed the things that concern vetting officers, focusing on the risks. We covered my life as a teenager, my family and friendship groups, gambling, drinking and prostitutes, as well as involvement with foreign nationals, places I'd been on holiday and some gentle questions about my current home life. But the questions seemed to lack the difficult probity I expected and we seemed close to the end of the interview ... and then, it came. 'Commander Jones [a compliment because I was in fact a lieutenant commander], I have listened to your very earnest questions about your life and reflecting upon your answers it seems most likely that you would not be the sort of officer who I would need to ask about their being involved with homosexuality. Is it correct that I need not ask you questions on that matter?' Despite my expectations, it was a bolt from the blue and I quickly analysed the question I'd been asked. Thinking as quickly as I could, it seemed that the question was 'Do I need to ask you about homosexuality?' No, he didn't – I was quite happy with my homosexuality! And so I replied, very simply, 'No sir, you don't.' 'Good,' he said. 'It's been a pleasure meeting you.' And he turned and left.

Years later, as a more senior officer, I realised that he knew. The vetting agency had unrestricted access to a wide range of documents as an enabler to their important work of making sure that defence secrets are safe. I had clearly been risk assessed ahead of the interview and deemed to have the integrity to be unbribable. On reflection, it was the beginnings of a change of heart at the MoD, but unable to see that, I simply breathed a puzzled sigh of relief and moved on with life.

And so, in the closing months of 1999, I was the perfect storm: a determined and gritty professional war fighter with an innate sense of justice who had watched ten years of denigration of duty and abandonment of the covenant by service chiefs. I had seen colleagues dismissed, outed and humiliated, and I had seen the careers

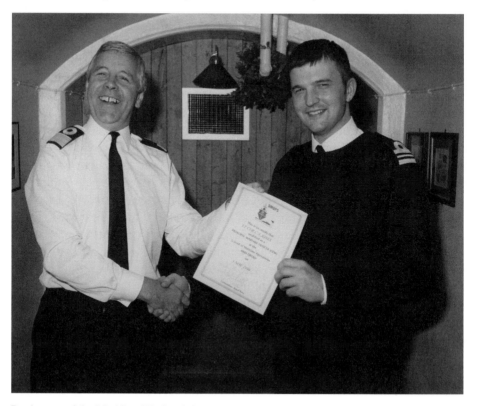

Passing out of the Maritime Warfare School as a 'Principal Warfare Officer' a few months after the vetting interview.

of talented servicemen and women lost. By then my confidential reports were once again positive, but damage had been done and I knew what injustice felt like. The time was coming when I would never again have to stand by in silence, and there was a fire in my soul that would not be put out. That fire had been kindled in a battle; the battle for the covenant was not over and I planned it would be won.

I wasn't always angry. At times, I was almost an apologist for an Armed Forces that, for a period of time, chose to set aside its core values. Before the ban was overturned and early in my career I almost convinced myself that it seemed reasonable that service chiefs might defend their long-held position. But as the years passed, good men and women were dismissed and the covenant was left behind. As I witnessed the damage being done, it became very clear that the day would come when I would draw my sword and charge, not in spite of my commission and duty, but because of it.

***

HMS *Fearless* was the grand old lady of the Fleet and at one time, command ship for land operations in the Falklands War, she had earned a place in the affections of thousands of servicemen and women across four decades. I was to join the ship as she ploughed her way up the Channel, bringing her deployment-weary crew ever closer to excited families and Christmas leave in her home port of Portsmouth.

Fearless had been on an exercise with a NATO Task Force for a few weeks and her return via the Channel provided an opportunity for me to have a couple of nights at sea with my fellow officers before taking over my new role. As soon as the ship was alongside in Portsmouth, the crew would scatter to all corners of the UK, and I wanted to get to know them – and for them to get to know me – as quickly as possible. Change was coming and time was running out for me.

Joining by a long helicopter ride in winter was not my preferred mode of transport, but after years of serving in aircraft carriers, I had become accustomed to the noisy, cold, draughty and somewhat uncomfortable experience. For the pilot and observer (navigator), there was a window to look out of, ear guards in a well-fitting safety helmet and a comfortable seat. However, in the back of the cab there was an air of austerity about this mode of travel.

The Royal Naval Air Station at Culdrose in Cornwall was the nearest landing site to the ship's planned route so I grabbed a hire car and headed down, with just a couple of olive green holdalls containing the basics of uniform and toiletries. There was something distinctly unmilitary about civvy suitcases and I had no wish to step onto the flight deck of my new ship trailing a Samsonite roller and looking like cabin crew. The officers' mess at Culdrose was home to 814 Squadron, 'The Flying Tigers', and 849 Squadron, with its airborne early warning capability, who spent much of their time embarked in the aircraft carriers. I was very much a 'carrier queen', a curious bit of naval slang for those of us who availed of the comforts of our larger aircraft carriers. The mess was busy with pilots and aircrew enjoying a last few days together before returning to their families for Christmas leave, and there were lots of familiar faces. It was a rule of thumb that after five years' service, you could walk into a wardroom anywhere in the Fleet and sit down for a beer with somebody you had served with. I was then in my eleventh year of service and knew that my evening would be spent remembering past deployments and visits to ports in far-flung parts of the world, and I joined a group of young aircrew with whom I had served in the Gulf in 1997. They had completed their last day of flying before Christmas and were loud and raucous, sat amidst a range of drinks that looked like somebody had raided a minibar. As I finished my second gin and tonic, I remembered a past two-hour helicopter flight to Bari in Italy on the morning after a Trafalgar Night Mess Dinner (the Royal Navy's annual commemoration of the death of Lord Nelson), and the thought of rattling around in a helicopter with a hangover again didn't appeal. So I turned in early amidst a barrage of raucous banter.

The following morning, I found myself in the crew room, looking out across the airfield at the grey Sea King helicopter that would take me to the ship. The sliding door was slammed shut behind me and I looked out across the apron towards the crew room. It looked inviting and I couldn't help but wonder if it might have been easier to meet my colleagues in Portsmouth!

I had always looked forward to joining a new ship, but this time was very different: life was about to change; there was no turning back. It was Wednesday, 8 December 1999, and two days before, while packing my holdalls, I had received the call from Angela Mason, Executive Director of Stonewall – the gay and lesbian equality charity. Stonewall had been fighting the gay ban for a decade and I'd kept in touch, always using telephone boxes or lines that could not be traced before checking in. By then I had high-level security clearance and had completed specialised training in signal intelligence gathering at GCHQ. I knew the risks of secure and insecure telephone lines and I had been extremely cautious over the years. As soon as I heard Angela's voice I knew what would follow: 'It's over, Craig,' she said, 'they're making an announcement early in the new year, in Parliament.' I had planned for this moment for many years, but the longer I served, the clearer it became that the services would struggle with this begrudged change and my first thoughts of a joyous day had given way over the years to an acceptance that I would simply exchange one complicated life for another.

12 January 2000: It was a little after 4.00 pm when the Right Honourable Geoff Hoon, Secretary of State for Defence, stood up to address the Commons. It had already been a long day and after lunch in the wardroom I had walked onto the upper deck to clear my head. The seamen were out painting the ship, a task that was never quite completed. I was still a new face, and I introduced myself to a number of the

men and women who were working 'up top' on this crisp and cold January day. Most had been home for Christmas leave, which made for easy conversation, and those who hadn't got home were eagerly looking forward to their break. I quipped the adage 'Second leave is best' with those who were yet to get away. After an hour or so, I returned to my cabin and slid shut the nearly 40-year-old metal door. In my cabin there was a sturdy wood-framed bunk, which folded back by day to provide a bench seat. Beside it there was a writing desk with shelves above and retaining straps to keep my warfare manuals and reference books in place in rough weather or at war. There was a wardrobe that was little more than torso high and closing the door needed both hands and the toe of my boot, ideally while listing to starboard so the suits swung away from the door. On my desk there was a large green blotter and a signal pad, upon which I wrote a wide range of classified 'signals' in an age before secure email found its place at sea. My bunk was folded back and had three broad leather straps to keep me in my bed in the worst of hurricanes. Tucked down the side there was a 'buggery board', which slotted into the middle of the bunk to brace against in the roughest sea states. Its name always reminded me

of the spirit and humour in the unique language of the Royal Navy and Royal Marines, a language that needs translating to family and friends for decades after completing your service. In my case, the buggery board saw little action because in a real storm I was always on the bridge. I had an iron stomach in the heaviest of blows and was always excited by a tumultuous sea. Driving a warship was the privilege of my life and I loved the seamanship challenge of keeping the ship steady in storm conditions. Learning the technicalities of the missile systems, gunnery and sonars needed to work in the operations room had been a struggle, but on the

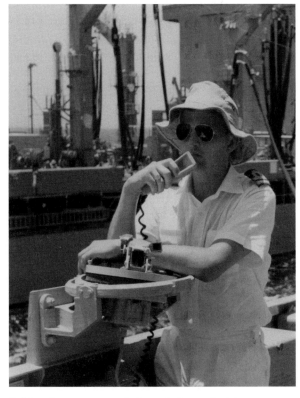

Driving from compass platform during replenishment at sea, one of the most hazardous evolutions a warship ever undertakes.

bridge of a ship I was in my element and I had an instinctive knowledge of the art of 'sea keeping'. I was always popular with our chefs, who faced the daily challenge of cooking three square meals a day (four in wartime) in heavy seas. Too fast running down the waves risked a broach, where the ship suddenly veered to be beam on to the rolling waves. In the worst cases, warships had rolled 70 degrees when knocked down by towering waves. Too slow and we risked being pooped (overrun by the towering waves). *Fearless* had a dock gate and an aircraft hangar at her stern, so pooping could cause very serious damage to our ability to launch and recover our Royal Marine Landing Craft or to the multi-million pound aircraft.

I was to take over the role of Operations Officer from Lieutenant Commander Peter Sparkes when he completed his tour later that month. Peter was a terrific officer, blessed with good humour and a gangly but athletic stature. He was also a gifted warfare officer, skilled at driving and fighting ships, and was highly respected and universally well liked. Our paths first crossed on our Officer of the Watch Course, where we learned our trade of driving warships in the gentlemanly countryside setting of HMS Mercury, in the stunningly beautiful Meon Valley in Hampshire. I was forever grateful to Peter for his help and encouragement to pass my Battle Fitness Test, a prerequisite of being able to continue the course. Peter recognised that I was a reluctant and unenthusiastic runner and he virtually pushed me around the course and over the line. It is these moments of camaraderie, teamwork and friendship in peacetime that form the bonds upon which we rely in war. Peter was an officer I would wish to go to war with, if we had to, and I was pleased and reassured to have him around in January 2000.

Peter had handed his cabin over to me early. It was larger and had extra seating space for meetings associated with my new role. Taking over as Head of Operations so soon after completing my year-long Principal Warfare Course was daunting. *Fearless* was a 'snake's wedding' of systems, bringing together a unique mix of a handful of modern self-defence capabilities with engineering, propulsion and domestic services systems that belonged in a museum. The weapons and marine engineering teams faced the daily challenge of keeping the old girl going by integrating systems that on any ordinary day were either incompatible or broken.

13 January 2000, 1552 hrs: In the corner of my cabin above my desk was a loudspeaker, thickly coated with almost forty years' worth of paint. Below the speaker was a Lego-style Bakelite volume switch and a tarnished brass on/off toggle. I sat on my bunk, flicked the toggle and cranked the switch around to hear the broadcast live from Parliament. The speaker crackled into life and I came in in mid-sentence to hear Jack Straw answering awkward questions about the ailing General Pinochet's convalescence in London. I flicked my cabin light off, to be alone in the dark with the crackly speaker and my thoughts. The continued presence of General Pinochet was an embarrassment and Mr Straw was no doubt pleased to give way to his fellow cabinet minister, the Secretary of State for

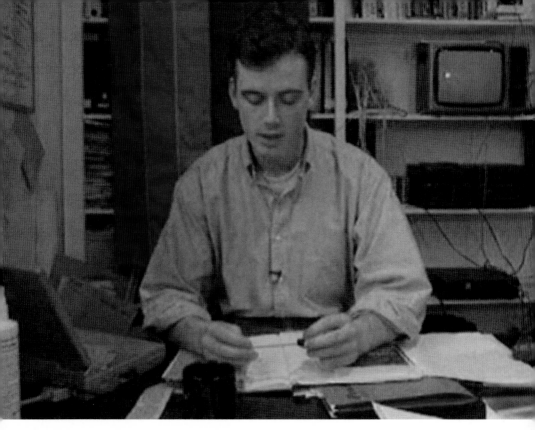

Above: *Sub Lt Edmund Hall RN, May 1995.*

Below: *Lt Cdr Patrick Lyster-Todd RN, Belize, 1985.*

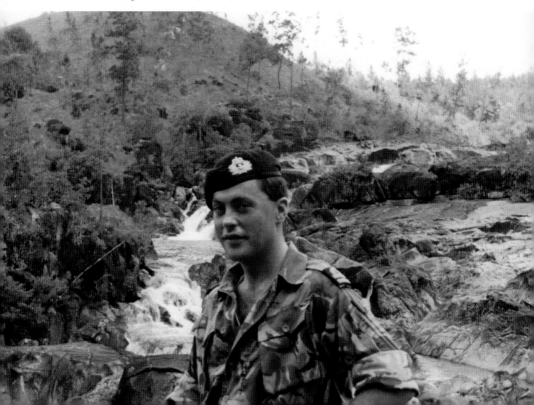

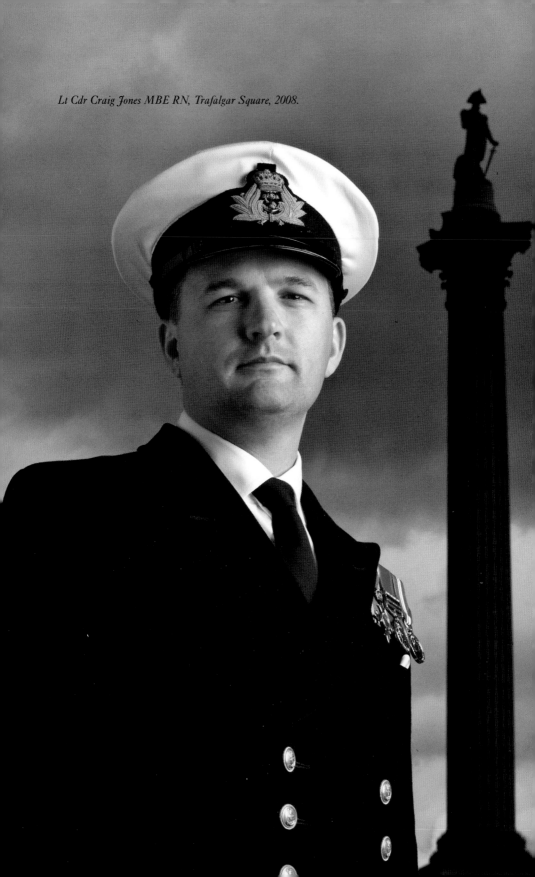

Lt Cdr Craig Jones MBE RN, Trafalgar Square, 2008.

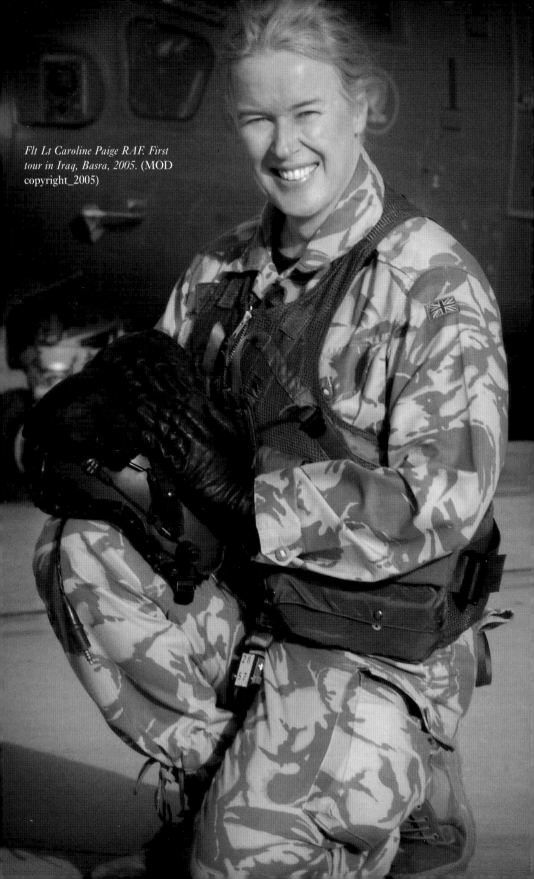

Flt Lt Caroline Paige RAF. First tour in Iraq, Basra, 2005. (MOD copyright_2005)

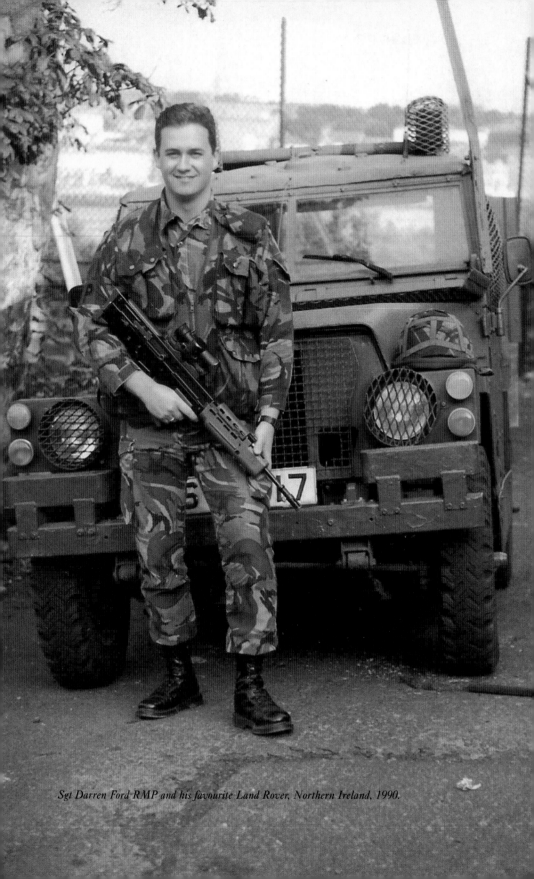

Sgt Darren Ford RMP and his favourite Land Rover, Northern Ireland, 1990.

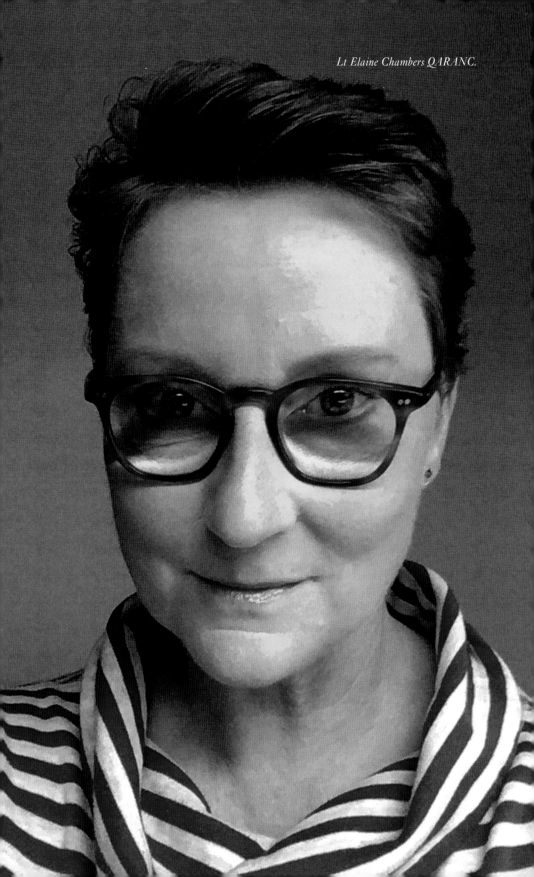

Lt Elaine Chambers QARANC.

Cdr Roly Woods RN, British Defence and Naval Attaché, pictured in Algiers Harbour in HMS Sheffield, 2002.

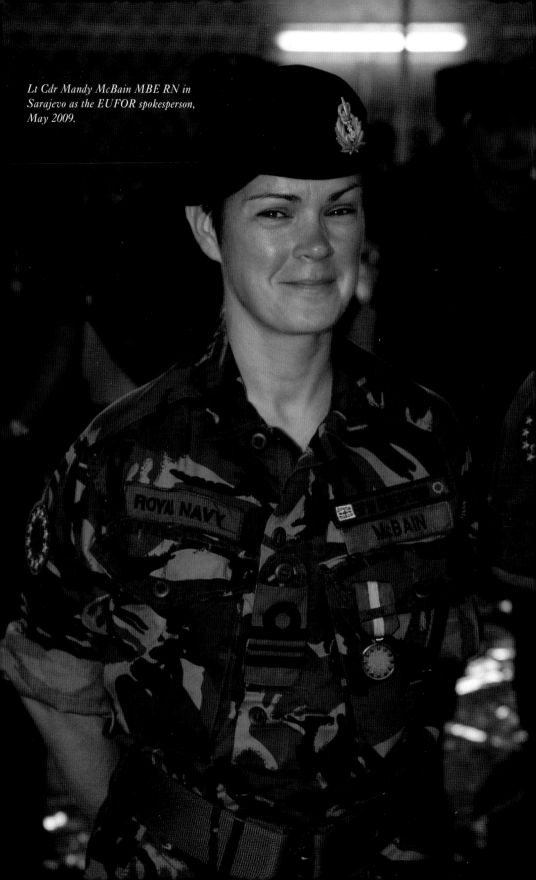

Lt Cdr Mandy McBain MBE RN in Sarajevo as the EUFOR spokesperson, May 2009.

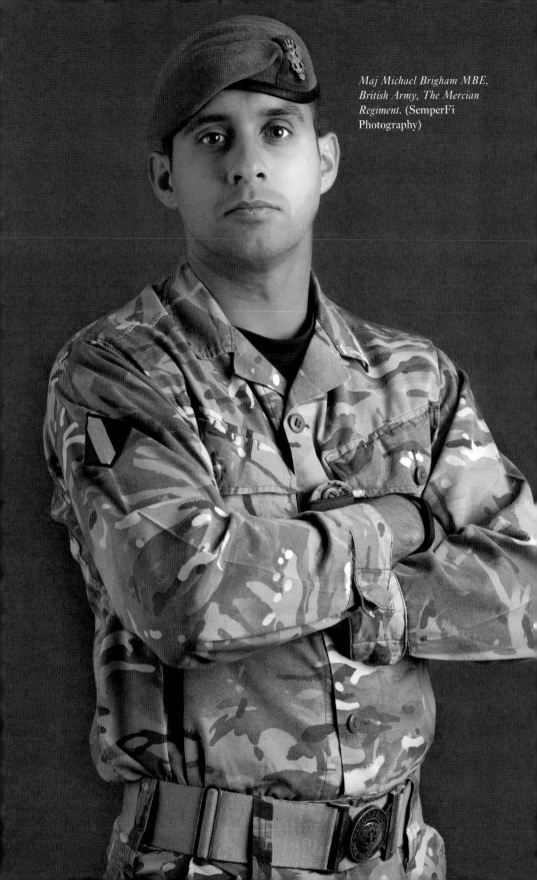

Maj Michael Brigham MBE, British Army, The Mercian Regiment. (SemperFi Photography)

Defence. Geoff Hoon stood up to begin a speech I had waited a very long time to hear, but the pause as Straw sat down and Hoon stood made me think that Hoon had been in no rush.

The greater part of Hoon's short speech focused upon the fact that the change of policy he was to announce was born of necessity, following a European Court of Human Rights ruling in September of the previous year. Lustig-Prean vs United Kingdom established that the ban on gay men and women serving in the UK Armed Forces was a breach of Article 8 of the Treaty of Maastricht, which identified the right to a private life. It was important that the case had been won; however, it was not a foregone conclusion that the UK would lift the ban, and there had been a long and difficult wait for news. The court's technical focus upon the link between the ruling and the concept of what defined a private life had left me wondering for some months if the UK would adopt a policy that copied the US 'Don't Ask, Don't Tell' policy. This policy, brought in by Bill Clinton as a compromise position, had resulted in more gay men and women being dismissed than the total ban that preceded it. Thankfully, the Ministry of Defence had no wish to be dragged through another decade of unwinnable court cases and they adopted the Australian model of a 'Code of Social Conduct', defining the way in which sailors, soldiers and airmen and women should respect each other. It was simple common sense; however, the prevalence of the word 'private' early in his speech made me fearful of a policy that 'Dare Not Speak Its Name'.

Hoon may have found comfort when in the presence of senior officers by the government being compelled to implement change, but to me it lacked moral courage. His speech had an air of apology and I winced and grimaced with each turn of phrase. He continued pressing his point, repeating the court's technical statement that sexual orientation was a 'private matter'. This was to be at the heart of the Armed Forces' way of managing what was seen as a highly challenging change. This was, of course, a policy born in a storm, an outcome of years of battle by the services' most senior officers. I often wondered if that time and effort could have been better used petitioning for improvements to the equipment desperately needed by our front-line troops throughout the 1990s. Was it naive or wrong to hope for a triumphant statement heralding great change? Naive or not, Hoon made a rueful and begrudged statement and I couldn't help but think that he had examined all other options over a period of months before rising to his feet in the Commons that day.

He continued:

> Implementing the changes successfully will be a challenge for leadership at all levels of the Armed Forces, but such challenges are not new and all three Services will be equal to the task. With the commitment which is in place from the very highest levels of the chain of command,

> I am confident that our Armed Forces will adapt to the change in the
> professional manner for which they are rightly held in the very highest
> regard. There will be those who would have preferred to continue to
> exclude homosexuals, but the law is the law. We cannot choose the
> decisions we implement. The status quo is simply not an option. The
> code of social conduct centres on the paramount need to maintain the
> operational effectiveness of the Armed Forces. I have no doubt it is the
> best way forward.

My cabin was dimly lit, but still I sat at my desk, head in my hands to shut out
the little light that prevailed. Were we really to announce a policy that bridged a
gaping hole in the Armed Forces Covenant by saying that 'the law is the law and
you cannot pick and choose'? Did we honestly believe that managing the continued
service of our remarkable gay servicemen and women would be challenging? I was
angry. Very angry.

The speech ended and other MPs rose to their feet to speak. A debate continued
and I zoned in and out. Ian Duncan Smith clearly lamented the change and there
seemed sympathy in his tone with Geoff Hoon's depiction of a Hobson's choice.
There were considerate and closed-minded statements and questions from across
the political divide, none of which mattered. With some relief, I listened to a
comment by Gerald Kaufman MP:

> Over the years, indeed centuries, homosexuals have served at every
> level in our Armed Forces with loyalty and distinction. Is it not better,
> therefore, to accept that fact than pretend it does not exist? It will not
> do for people to say that they oppose discrimination on the grounds
> of sexual orientation in principle when they act differently in practice.

This went to the very heart of the matter for me. I was appalled by the breach
of the Armed Forces Covenant and to this day, feel that a profound apology by
those in uniform who presided over this denigration of the fundamental duty of
officers has been missing. The covenant is a 'promise' made by the government
and those who have power and influence over our Armed Forces that those who
serve or have served, and their families, are treated fairly. It is not a new concept
and has existed in one form or another for over 400 years. A great deal of work
was done after 2000 to define the covenant, notably by General Sir Richard
Dannatt, later Chief of the General Staff of the Army. In the last few years of
my career I drew my sword repeatedly against General Dannatt and his staff.
However, I note with great respect that he believed that the men and women of
the Armed Forces were deserving of the corporate protection of our most senior
officers. My only criticism would be that for a few years, he left some of those men

and women behind because they were gay. Nevertheless, this honourable officer, with a strong Christian faith, earned my admiration and trust for unexpectedly doubling back, a matter I shall return to. As he stood up to speak, Geoff Hoon knew beyond question that thousands of serving gay men and women would hear his words. These stoic folk were already doing their ordinary duty in their ships, regiments and squadrons across the world, despite being corporately unwelcome for every day of their service leading to this day and for many days to come. The Ministry of Defence's treatment of these men and women had been shameful and the recalcitrance in Hoon's words and tone of his speech was not bringing those days to an end; it was continuing the hurt.

For a few moments, in my darkness, I felt lonely. There were of course people in society that had at the heart of their beliefs a clear understanding of the fact that it was nonsense to expect our Armed Forces to protect the ordinary freedoms that we had then denied them. But in January 2000, there was a prevailing majority view in Whitehall, and specifically in the Ministry of Defence, that hounding gay men and women out of the services had been in the country's best interests, and if they had been able to 'pick and choose', as Mr Hoon suggested, they would have done so.

My thoughts drifted to what the coming weeks would bring; some of this I knew, some could not be known. When I tuned back in to the parliamentary broadcast, Tam Dalyell, the MP for Linlithgow, was lamenting that he had attended a debate about Serbia earlier that afternoon in Westminster Hall and that the hall was stuffy, smelly and airless, and he compared the odour to a rather full school pupils' changing room. I rose to my feet and clicked the loudspeaker switch one turn to the left; that was enough of that. I grabbed my mobile phone and left my cabin, bound for the upper deck. It was time to call Matthew.

If there was one comfort on that day, it lay in the consistency of my viewpoint over the years of my service. My world and the service were converging, but the pace was always too slow for me. From the very beginnings of my time in the Royal Navy, I had found it very odd that an organisation at the heart of protecting our peace and freedoms should so irrationally accept a business case for a policy of exclusion that had more holes than a colander. My mind drifted back to where it all began ... with Michael Ball.

13 February 2000, 1800 hrs, Wardroom, HMS *Fearless*: The best I can say of my commanding officer in HMS *Fearless* would be that our views on the repeal of the gay ban were at variance. For me, the lifting of the ban was a blessed relief from living half my life in the shadows. It brought me back into the military family and restored my integrity, something fundamental to the service of an officer. My new commanding officer lamented being let down by 'the mandarins in Whitehall'. The year ahead would have its lively moments and I was never far from controversy. I came out in my commanding officer's cabin, to stem what

I saw as a denigration of the ordinary responsibility of officers to lead. Whether or not the change in policy was liked, it was our shared duty to implement it. This was the first opportunity for the covenant to be recognised for this beleaguered group and I was determined that the men and women in my ship would detect no hint of chagrin in the announcement that was to be made to them ahead of Geoff Hoon's speech to the Commons. My tactic worked and my commanding officer gave a deadpan address to the ship's company a few hours ahead of the formal announcement. But my stance set us up for an uneasy relationship, and I suspect we were both happy to part company early in the following year as I moved to a new role at HMS Collingwood.

What was truly remarkable about my time in HMS *Fearless* was that with each day that passed, the welcome of my ship's company grew warm and for the first time in my life, I truly felt part of the team. People work better when they can be themselves. Adam and I had waited a long time for the ban to be lifted and no moment was to be wasted. When the notice went up for a wardroom ball at the Queen's Hotel in Portsmouth to celebrate Burns Night on Saturday, 29 January, less than three weeks after the ban was lifted, I signed my name on the list and placed Adam's in the partner's box alongside it. What followed was a mix of delight from close colleagues and tangible panic from a small group of senior officers led by the Captain that seemed to focus upon whether Adam and I would dance together. I found this quite bizarre. As an officer, the dignity of the uniform is paramount, and never more so than in the company of partners. The idea of Adam and I dancing around the floor in some sort of 'gliding embrace' was a truly ridiculous notion, but it reflected the concern of a small cohort of officers across the service who perhaps considered notions such as whether gay officers might incorporate feather boas into their uniform to add a hint of pizzazz. I have often said that if held to the light, my watermark and defining characteristic is 'Royal Navy' and not 'gay', and I believe many of my brethren see the world similarly. It is our loyalty to the service that defines us.

Conscious that eyes would be upon Adam far more than on me, it was time to visit Gieves & Hawkes. From their base at No. 1 Savile Row, since 1771, 'Gieves' has won the affection of generations of Royal Navy officers for a classic English style that is instantly recognisable and has dressed kings and princes. No green bow ties or crimson cummerbunds, or shirts fit for Charles Aznavour's wardrobe; just simple, elegant gentlemen's clothes. They did their job, but I have to say that walking into the Queen's Hotel as the first gay partner to attend a formal function with a serving officer took raw courage and a great deal of dignity. Adam's dance card kept him busy all evening and if I'd wanted to take his hand in the ceilidh, I'd have had to join the queue. At a time when most officers didn't know what a gay partner looked like, Adam looked reassuringly like them. Not all courage is that of the battlefield.

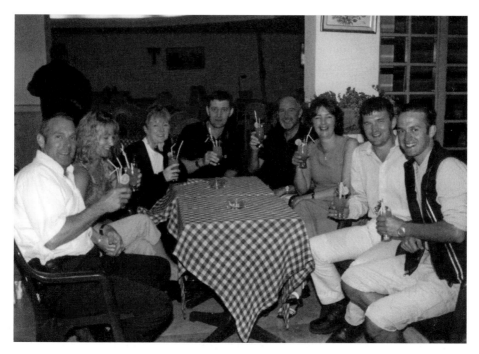

A run ashore in Turkey with officers, their wives and Adam, 2001.

In the years the followed, I continued to find my place in the service but was constantly aware of the difficulties being faced by other LGBTQ service personnel. By 2001, I was the Vice-Chair of the newly formed Armed Forces Lesbian and Gay Association and involved with an unduly reserved initiative by the personnel directorates to engage with LGBTQ personnel. Bullying, harassment and, in some cases, assault were far too common occurrences and there had been no effort at all to overturn the climate impact of a thirty-year strongly defended gay ban. My petitioning for change fell on deaf ears and I became increasingly angry that conservative attitudes from senior officers were setting the pace of change to the detriment of some of our most vulnerable personnel. In consequence, I undertook a range of initiatives to address an inclusive policy 'that dare not speak its name'. These were not welcome interventions and I found myself commonly at loggerheads with very senior officers who had a habit of writing to me, signing in the traditional green ink, to tell me how disappointed they were at having to admonish me (because I'd been vocal about the plight of gay colleagues or paid scant attention to Queen's Regulations and written directly to the Minister for the Armed Forces or the Secretary of State for Defence). In one exchange it was reported to me that a senior officer had said it was perfectly ordinary and no issue to be gay. I sent him an impertinent email and invited him to go to his local paper shop and buy a copy of *Gay Times* and post it to me though the internal mail system, if it were true that we lived in such a utopian society. I called his executive assistant a week later to be told that the Commodore had 'given it a go' without succeeding, and that the point had been well made. In June 2005, I snuck in through the back door of the Second Sea Lord's Diversity Conference, an event that welcomed over 100 captains of industry for presentations and a Q&A session. At the end, when the Q&A started, with the Royal Navy's head of personnel (Second Sea Lord) on stage, I asked why this prestigious event had passed with discussions about race, faith, ethnicity, gender, disability … indeed, every protected characteristic other than sexual orientation. The question won me another letter signed in green ink!

I have no idea about the role of luck in my life or whether the likes of Quentin Crisp or Oscar Wilde have sat on a cloud sprinkling fairy dust where it's most needed. However, there have been a handful of occasions when the turn of events has pulled me, bedraggled, from the lion's mouth.

With my latest green ink signed letter still smarting, I put my best uniform on and set off on the Saturday following the diversity conference to Trooping the Colour. Adam and I had won tickets in a lottery for military personnel, and it was a welcome distraction. Adam had kitted himself with morning dress for the occasion and I have to say, we looked quite dapper, but the air for me hung heavy with what had become all too regular clashes with service chiefs regarding their lack of positive message about their LGBTQ servicemen and women. But I dusted myself down for the occasion and we took our seats. In the course of the event I caught up with Lieutenant Polly McCowen, a logistics officer whom I had taught navigation in HMS *Fearless*. She was with her parents, who I remembered had some sort of association with the Civil Service. At the end of the pageantry they kindly hosted us for lunch at Leith's and during the discussions, my disappointment at the Armed Forces' lack of initiative for its LGBTQ community poured out. Polly's father was a distinguished man who I was later to establish was the Cabinet Secretary to the Thatcher government, Lord Armstrong of Ilminster, and perhaps one of the most important political figures of the second half of the twentieth century. Lady Armstrong sensed Polly's disquiet at my situation and by the end of the lunch it was evident that there was compassion for my invidious position.

A few days later, an invitation dropped onto our doormat that was to provide the breakthrough I had been unable to find in my petitioning of captains, commodores, vice admirals, generals, air marshals and ministers. The invite was to a private gathering at Leeds Castle, two nights over a weekend, when opera was being performed in the grounds for a wider audience. We arrived in our clapped-out Rover 216 to a scene reminiscent of *Upstairs Downstairs*, as staff whisked away our luggage (and our car even faster). The first meal was to be lunch and we changed to 'dog robbers' (naval slang for jacket and tie). As we left our room in one of the castle's turrets, we turned a corner and found ourselves face to face with First Sea Lord, Admiral Sir Alan West and Lady West. A little startled, I introduced myself by military rank and turned to introduce my boyfriend 'Adam'. Slightly mischievously, I accentuated the 'boy' bit, but without necessity; Lady West was brimming with delight at the encounter and I saw little more of Adam that weekend!

Over those fateful couple of days, I had the chance, in those uniquely private circumstances, to defend the corner of a group of servicemen and women who were deserving of the loyalty of service chiefs. Their loyalty had been unstinting, amidst circumstances that in many cases had been pretty awful, and Admiral West very clearly understood that. By the fall of the cards or aided by that sprinkling of fairy dust, I had stepped aside of all of the officers who had stood between me and the head of the Royal Navy, and my relief was dewy-eyed.

In the months that followed, Admiral West agreed changes that made a profound difference. With his support we were given the Military Chaplaincy at Amport for a weekend retreat to meet with senior officers. A signal was sent to every unit in the Armed Forces asking them to release anybody who wished to attend and to provide travelling expenses. It was a remarkable weekend, which brought together sixty LGBTQ personnel, every one of them moved and bewildered to be in the presence of so many of their kind. Lady 'Rosie' West remained a strong supporter and was on rare occasions a way to get a message to the First Sea Lord without my skipping through too many links in the chain of command. Admiral West set a new unabashed tone for supporting LGBTQ initiatives, which was followed by his successor, a face from my past, Admiral Sir Jonathan Band. On his watch I requested permission for our servicemen and women to march in uniform at Pride in London that summer. Chief of the General Staff of the Army and the Chief of the Air Staff flatly refused, and with some reluctance agreed that polo shirts with military crests might be used. I very strongly made the point that service personnel do not march in polo shirts in public; our uniform is our second skin. Thankfully, Admiral Band agreed. It was one of those occasions when the balance of risk and reward was not good. The reward was to do the right thing; the risk was to have the Naval Service embarrassed in the world press, just a few weeks following embarrassing press coverage of the kidnap of Royal Navy personnel in the Gulf. In the footsteps of Admiral West, I felt that Admiral Band had been brave, and it needed to go well. Working with the MoD Press Office, I called every gay hack in Fleet Street. The story that followed was reported in every world news title from the *Sydney Morning Herald* to the *San Francisco Bay Chronicle*. There was not one dissenting article, and all were accompanied by remarkable images of those marching. In the weeks that followed, I was told that the Secretary of State asked why the British

Army and Royal Air Force had sent their personnel to a public event at which they marched in civilian clothing. It is in many ways a pity that Admiral Band and I never crossed paths with time for the 'fireside chat' that might have lain to rest the ghosts of HMS *Illustrious*. However, when in full knowledge of the facts, he had taken the right fork in the road.

Even as late as 2006 and 2007, there were pockets of resistance, and General Dannatt, Chief of the General Staff, briefly became a focus (now General the Lord Dannatt). On a couple of occasions I leaked his position on LGBTQ issues to *The Sunday Times*, specifically about the General being reported as 'apoplectic about being pushed by ministers to allow the Army to march in uniform at Pride'. Leaking to the press is a poor behaviour, but I had no other mechanism with which to address an issue with such a senior officer. By the end of 2007, I had gathered from the General's office that he had experienced an epiphany and was now very positive about his LGBTQ personnel, so I desisted in my campaign. Before departing the service in May 2008, I requested a leaving call with General Dannatt. It was an unusual ask from a relatively junior Royal Navy officer, but he accepted my request. In our meeting he very earnestly told me that he had changed his view. Knowing that he had a strong faith, which might have caused him conflict, I thanked him for the support he had shown of late and left him with a challenge: to give the opening address in the Armed Forces LGBTQ Conference to be hosted by the Army in the following October, noting that I would not be there to leak to the press whether he had done it or not. The speech he made was reported to me as being very moving for those who attended, underpinned by this distinguished officer's understanding of the fundamental importance of the covenant. I am always impressed by allies who support our community, because an understanding of the business case is in their DNA. I am slightly more impressed by those for whom this is a struggle from the outset, but one that they overcome.

The chance to do my duty was won by veterans who fought for change such that my career might not be dashed. When the ban was lifted, I did not turn my back on their support but instead turned my head towards the job of making the new policy work. I hope that my fellow veterans now understand that necessity.

Sometimes I wonder if there are senior officers or colleagues who feel I owe them an apology. There were certainly LGBTQ colleagues who winced at my unmilitary approach to this campaign, which at times verged on insubordination. Many of those struggling to find their way after the ban was lifted were keen to pass quietly in their daily military lives, but so many more needed the Armed Forces to pick up the baton. There is undoubtedly a generation of senior officers who rolled their eyes at the thought of the antics of the 'unsinkable' Craig Jones.

Today, I am thankful for the chance I was given to do my duty in the only way I know how. Nobody need ever ask me what I did during the war! These days, though, I check if a door is open before I break it down.

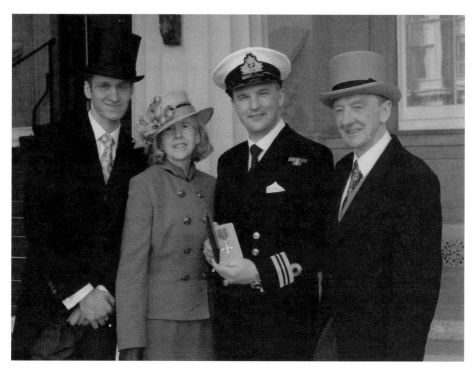

Buckingham Palace, 2007, with my parents, and Adam in a tall top hat!

'Gay in the Armed Forces', by Craig Jones,
New Statesman, 28 July 2008

As Geoff Hoon announced the repeal of the UK Armed Forces 'gay ban' on 13th January 2000, just a few yards down the road there were long faces in the Ministry of Defence.

The repeal of the 'gay ban' was a critically important win for equality campaigners and heralded the beginnings of Blairite social changes which have made the UK a far better place for gay men and women to be. But be in no doubt, it was not welcomed by many in the British military establishment.

My Commanding Officer told a packed Officers' Mess of the policy change a day before the House of Commons announcement and we were all placed under strict embargo. My response was swift and instinctive; I stepped from my closet and claimed the ground which had been so hard fought for.

Secrecy and deceit go against the grain of the often-enduring friendships that we enjoy in the Armed Forces. My ship's company seemed to recognise that my choice of openness set me on a difficult path and after a bewildering first week, I felt their growing support.

I cannot think of a civilian life equivalent to the 'band of brothers' atmosphere that exists in the wardroom of a warship. And it was profoundly rewarding to see attitudes and ideas about being gay change over time.

Yet beyond the few units who won themselves an 'out' guy or girl, in Whitehall the MoD fumbled around and achieved little for a number of years at substantial cost to a courageous group of junior ranks who took the difficult path of being open.

At times I have defended my kind like a tiger and as I depart the service it's timely to acknowledge that there is a group of wounded senior officers who have received acerbic letters, emails or – far worse – a visit from me over the years. The fact that I have escaped 'jankers' makes me think that they took my unmilitary directness with a pinch of 'sea salt' – a faint heart never won a fair maiden. It's sometimes difficult to tell the difference between those who have insight and those who are simply incensed; on most occasions I feel I had a little of both. Nevertheless I suspect that admirals, generals and air marshals have traded my letters in the gentlemen's clubs of London.

The exception was Admiral Lord West of Spithead, now minister for internal security. His unstinting early support for the gay community in the Armed Forces paved the path others would later follow when the shrapnel stopped flying. His successor, Admiral Sir Jonathan Band, has matched his initiative despite the occasional recalcitrance of other services.

So eight years on as the British Army joins Stonewall's good employers scheme and gay sailors, soldiers and air folks march through London with swords drawn and shiny medals, clapped and cheered by an adoring crowd – has this social experiment worked? Gay men and women are now serving with pride and distinction alongside their heterosexual colleagues at the front line of operations worldwide. They enjoy increasing levels of support from their command and service chiefs and the Armed Forces no longer dismiss highly trained and much-needed personnel. A few months after Gulf War II, I chatted to a gay soldier about his experiences of being at the front line and with a cheeky grin he lamented that his fellow infantrymen seemed 'far more interested in invading Iraq than me and my sexual orientation – but who knows, they might ask me to go back and redecorate!' It occurred to me that I was talking to the man for whom Rank Outsiders had fought so hard.

Gay servicemen and women of my generation will always be indebted for their courage and enduring fortitude to win equality and justice for the Armed Forces of today.

Reprinted by kind permission of *New Statesman*

Chapter 4

Homosexuality in the Armed Forces
A memorandum submitted by
Captain Professor Sir Michael Howard OM CH MC
British Army Coldstream Guards

Michael Howard is not new to battle, being one of a dwindling number of our Second World War veterans. He joined the Coldstream Guards in 1942 and after a period of training he deployed through North Africa and fought in the Italian Campaign, with the 3rd Battalion, coming ashore during the landings in Salerno in September 1943. During his first engagement with the enemy he was awarded the Military Cross, a medal he accepted noting that he felt there were more worthy candidates.

Later in his career, Sir Michael was to become Regius Professor of Modern History at Oxford and is considered one of the United Kingdom's greatest living historians.

To gay men and women in the Armed Forces he epitomises our elder brethren and it is no surprise that in 1995 he picked up his pen, as he might have picked up his sword earlier in his career. In a memorandum sent at this critical point in the battle for equality in the Armed Forces, he wrote to the Permanent Under Secretary of the day making a compelling case for change.

In our band of brothers (and sisters) Michael Howard stands tall and we shall always be grateful for his testament in defence of both the shared values of the Armed Forces and of the covenant.

Dear Sir,

I have asked leave to present this memorandum since I believe that I am one of the few people in this country equally familiar with the world of the Armed Forces and with that of the 'homosexual community'. More important, I am in the fortunate position of being able to say so quite frankly.

My knowledge of the Armed Forces is based not so much on my own experience as an infantry officer fifty years ago, in a large National Service army very different from the small and highly professional services of today, as on the close relationship I have maintained with all three services in the past forty years: as an adviser on educational policy and organisation, and as a lecturer at service colleges at every level from cadet colleges to the Royal College of Defence Studies. I have also enjoyed the friendship, and the close confidence, of several generations of senior officers, some of whom indeed were my pupils at Oxford.

My knowledge of the world of homosexuals comes from inside. I am myself homosexual and enjoy the company of a wide range of homosexual friends. All are honest, honourable, hardworking and patriotic people, many of whom have achieved great distinction in their professions.

My service experience, both at first and at second-hand, makes me understand very well why homosexuals present problems to the Armed Forces. I assume that no one needs to argue that homosexuals of either sex are likely to be any less courageous, reliable and efficient at their jobs than their heterosexual colleagues; any such arguments are easily confuted by the factual record of the Second World War. Nor are homosexuals in the Armed Forces any more likely to make unwanted sexual advances to members of their own sex than are heterosexuals to the opposite. If such cases do occur they are clear breaches of military discipline and can be dealt with as such.

I suggest, therefore, that the problem arises primarily from the social unacceptability of known homosexuals in units where combat efficiency depends on a mutual understanding and comradeship of like-minded people who share common values and – it must be said – common prejudices. In groups that set a high value on 'masculinity' and whose life revolves, while young, around the pursuit of girls and, when older, around the problems of married life, homosexuals do not easily fit. Those who display their sexual orientations by their actions or behaviour are likely – unless they have exceptional countervailing qualities – to be 'extruded from the herd' whatever official policy may be on the matter. Arguments drawn from the examples of classical Greece or Sparta, or even from front-line experiences in two world wars, will cut little ice in the sergeants' or petty officers' mess. Commanding officers may dislike such prejudices, but they have to tolerate them. Their job is to run efficient units, not schools for politically correct behaviour. Nevertheless, if they do allow themselves to be affected by such prejudices, they may deprive them of the services of some first-rate soldiers.

A lifetime of experience has shown me, however, that homosexuals are infinitely diverse, and cannot be stereotyped. For many, their sexual inclination is the least significant element of their personalities. Homosexuals come in all different shapes and sizes. Among them are to be found large numbers of happy and respected schoolteachers, nurses, academics, administrators and indeed servicemen, able to make a unique contribution to the communities that they serve. Such people do not consider themselves to belong to the 'homosexual community'; they belong to their own communities, whether schools, colleges, hospitals, villages, churches or, given the chance, the Armed Forces, and they can bring to them special qualities of dedication.

To arbitrarily exclude such people from the opportunity of serving in the Armed Forces is not so much unjust as contrary to the best interests of the Armed

Forces themselves, especially in times of difficult recruitment. They have an enormous contribution to make. It is illogical to deny people the opportunity of serving in the Armed Forces for no other reason than that they are not attracted to the opposite sex.

People should not be penalised or punished for what they are, but for what they do. Unless the Armed Forces recognise this, their practice will be at variance, not only with that of all other organisations in this country, including the fire service and the police, but in conflict with enduring ethical values for which this country is supposed to stand and has fought several wars in this century to uphold.

Yours Faithfully,
Michael Howard

Chapter 5

My Life as the First Openly Serving Transgender Officer in the British Armed Forces

Flight Lieutenant Caroline Paige

Royal Air Force

My career in the military began on a winter's day in January 1980. I already held a private pilot's licence, thanks to winning an RAF flying scholarship as an air cadet at school, so it seemed natural that the Royal Air Force became my choice of service, even though I grew up with the Army, where my father had been a staff sergeant in the Royal Artillery.

My first posting following training was to a fighter squadron in Scotland, as a navigator on No. 111 (F) Squadron, flying the F4 Phantom. The Cold War was in full swing and our role was air defence of the United Kingdom and her NATO allies. To the east, the Warsaw Pact had the capability for a pre-emptive strike and we had to be ready for that. Arms controls and diplomatic conversation, along with the deterrent of the devastating consequences of war between nuclear armed super powers, was enough to keep the peace, but it was a delicate peace, and one we had to be prepared to defend and deter from being broken.

The Phantom was an extraordinary aeroplane with an international pedigree, a 58-foot long, 25-ton aircraft, carrying two crew, eight air-to-air missiles and a Gatling gun, and capable of flying almost twice the speed of sound. Its state-of-the-art look-down/shoot-down radar helped make it the most capable all-round fighter interceptor that the UK had in the Cold War period. Because of a ground-based early warning radar capability and the speed of the aircraft, it was more practical and economical to have aircraft holding an alert status on the ground ready to scramble airborne fully armed. This was known as Quick Reaction Alert (Intercept) or QRA(I), where aircrew on a twenty-four-hour rotation, and ground crew sharing week-long duties, ate, slept and worked in a small detached building beside the aircraft, with a commitment to get at least one fighter airborne as soon as possible, any time of the day or night and in all weathers. The Soviet Union played its part in all of this, too, regularly testing

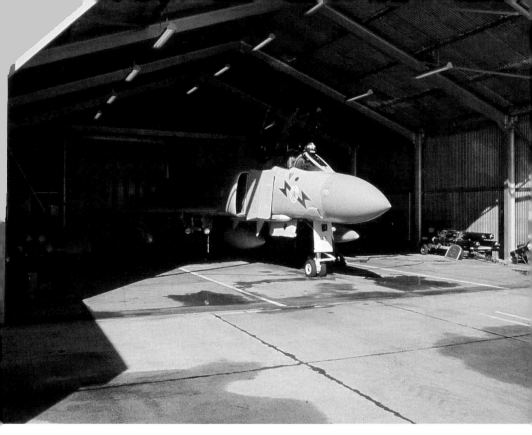

Above and below: Holding Quick Reaction Alert, and up close with a Soviet 'Bear' west of the Faroe Islands, RAF Leuchars, 1986.

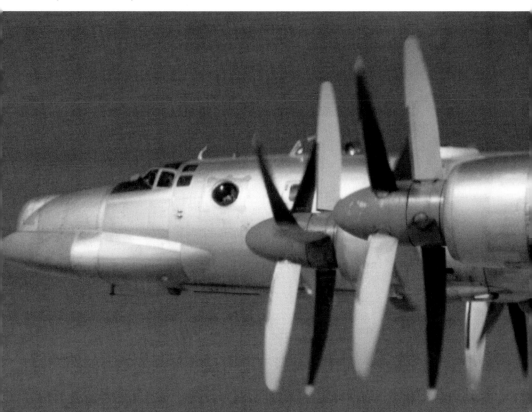

our defensive responses and reaction times with their long-range bombers, seeking to capture and exploit any weaknesses. During my seven years at RAF Leuchars, I intercepted a total of thirty-four Bears, a giant four-engine contra-rotating propeller-driven bomber, used for many different roles, including nuclear strike.

Our daily task was to train for war, because tomorrow might be too late. 'Train as you fight' it was known as, and we exercised our skills day and night, in diverse environments and conditions. But training for war in representative scenarios pushed aircrew and aircraft to the limits, and several colleagues and good friends were killed in tragic accidents doing so. For every crew lost there were many more where luck just happened to be on their side, perhaps for a split second, but that would be the difference between life or death. It was the nature of military flying in the 1980s: it was the 'work hard' side of the coin, and the reason there was a 'play hard' social balance. It was challenging flying, and I experienced many 'luck moments'. A crash-landing at RAF Akrotiri in Cyprus saw our aircraft damaged beyond economic repair; another accident saw us crash 800 feet across a Kent field at a 100mph, after a brake malfunction while landing at Biggin Hill, and there were many more times my heart missed a beat. It was an amazing job, though, and I was proud of my achievements.

Yet living this 'top gun' existence couldn't have been any more different from my life up until then. I had been hiding a secret for nearly twenty years … one that would bring a hard fall with no mercy if discovered. My family, friends and country were proud of me, but I knew that pride would be revoked the moment they learned the truth that within me was a voice that wouldn't be tolerated, that couldn't be heard, that was too scared of the consequences. My secret was gender identity, because although I had been identified male at birth, my soul identified as female. I didn't understand how that could be. My earliest recollections of questioning my gender identity start from the age of 5: a memory burned into my little brain when my father caught me wearing one of my sister's dresses and made it absolutely clear that it was wrong, that it was queer, that it was shameful … abnormal … pathetic, even. Boys were boys, and girls were girls; there were clear boundaries. Yet every message coming from my young brain was saying I was right, that he was wrong. I could only imagine that every other person knew who they were with equal conviction, but they never had reason to question their gender. Why would they? Fortunately for them, their instincts were supported by visual assurance: the very fabric of their being was male or female, and the body they had reinforced that. My body didn't match my soul. It was my sex that was wrong, not my gender, and because I knew of no way to resolve that, or prove it, I had to hide it away, and my life became an essential masquerade.

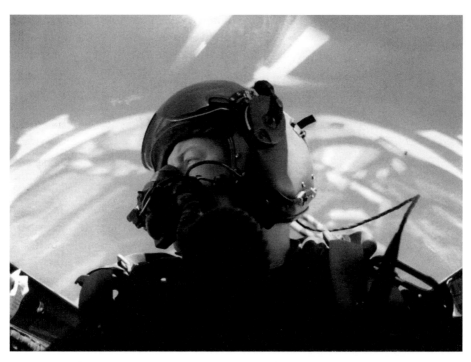

F4 cockpit, 1987: This 'top gun' existence couldn't have been any more different from my life up until then.

My career gave me the opportunity for my own space, somewhere away from all those expectations, somewhere my secret didn't have to hide so much. It gave me the ability to buy a house of my own; a safe environment that allowed me to be the opposite of the image everyone saw, that everyone expected, that everyone demanded. I couldn't afford to let anyone see that, because I was in the military now, and as far as the military of the day was concerned, lesbian, bisexual and transgender individuals were gay, and military law forbade gay service.

Although I knew I wasn't gay, nobody understood what being transgender meant; even *I* hadn't heard the word in public use. Discovery would bring instant dismissal, harassment, intimidation and outing, regardless of the implications that might have on someone who had not yet 'come out' to family or friends. Dismissal from service would be 'conduct unbecoming', 'not needed for service' or 'without honour', irrespective of that person's likely exemplary service. I knew the military even had its own investigative teams, responding to 'rumour' as much as evidence, and they often did that in the most invasive, humiliating and inhuman way. I not only saw and heard what happened to those who were discovered or outed in this way, but service personnel were also encouraged to report 'signs of

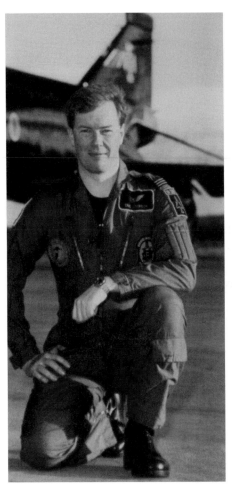

Formal photo with F4 Phantom *Black Mike* on 111 (F) Squadron, 1989. (*MoD Copyright 1989*)

homosexual behaviour'. People were discriminated against in the most awful of ways even though they were serving their own country, with all the accepted risk to life that that entailed. Secrecy was the key to survival, and so I led a double life, worried that any clues to my gender identity would bring everything crashing down.

The fact that I lived this way for so long without discovery was testament to just how hard I worked at not being discovered. I think the scale of opposites did afford me some protection: my visible life as 'top gun' aircrew flying an amazing aircraft in as macho an environment as there could possibly be; and my invisible life where I needed everything to be reassuringly feminine. However, the biggest worry by far was losing my family. I already knew their opinions, and as much as that prevented me from being true to myself, I still loved them, and I didn't want my actions to destroy them, as I knew it would. Having achieved a commission had made them proud, but that pride was in the person they knew, not the person I was; I was living to their expectations, and those of my colleagues, service and society. Revealing such an intimate part of my own life spelt disaster: without a job there was no home, without family and friends there was no support, without societal acceptance there was no future.

***

In November 1989, my time with the F4 Phantom came to an end and I was posted to No. 63 Squadron at RAF Chivenor, in North Devon, flying the Hawk in a tactical training role. The Hawk was a tandem-seat jet trainer, and our role was to teach student fast-jet pilots and navigators the difference between flying an aircraft and operating it. We were teaching them the fighting skills, tactics, crew cooperation and basic weapons knowledge they needed before graduating to operational aircraft such as Phantom, Tornado, Harrier, Jaguar and Buccaneer. The squadron also had a war role called Mixed Fighter Force, where we flew the Hawk in short-range defence of assets in the United Kingdom, joining with the larger air defence fighters or protecting allocated sites, from airfields to cities. When I arrived in Chivenor, the Cold War was still very much the operational focus, but times were changing and the Iron Curtain dividing Eastern and Western Europe was crumbling.

On the evening of the 1990 Summer Bank Holiday Monday, the phone rang at my parents' house, where I was enjoying a spot of leave and eating dinner. Within twelve hours I was sat in an RAF C-130 Hercules, heading to a possible war. Saddam Hussein had invaded Kuwait, and sixteen hours after leaving RAF Lyneham, I disembarked at an airbase called Dhahran, in Saudi Arabia's Eastern Province. I had never seen so many combat aircraft in my life – far more, it seemed, than we had in the whole RAF inventory. We learned we were part of Operation Granby – or Desert Shield, as the US called their operational deployment – a huge response from multinational forces rapidly building up to help deter any further Iraqi aggression. This would be my home for a yet undetermined period.

Providing air attack practice for a RN ship in a Hawk T.Mk1A, English Channel, 1991.

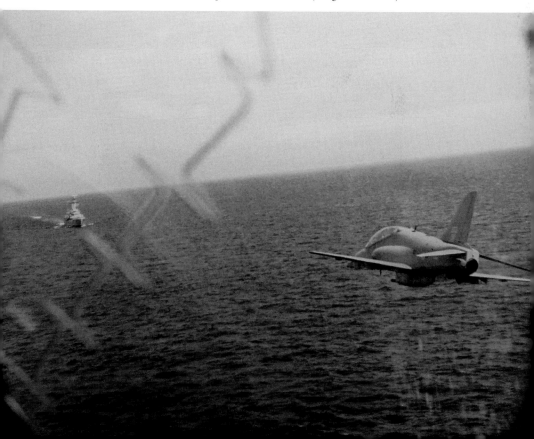

The possibility of being in a war didn't worry me. If the worst happened, then my lifetime worries would be over. It wasn't that I didn't want to live. I had considered ending my days more often than I cared to remember, but ending my life because of what others thought or expected seemed senseless: I lost, they won. So war didn't worry me, but I certainly respected the danger I could be in. Over the next few months we prepared for defensive operations, and for attack, should that be the outcome of failed political negotiation. I worked as an operations officer in the Tactical Air Operations Centre at Dhahran, covering UK fast-jet operations in the operational area. We were always armed, due to the risk of kidnap or terrorist action off-base, and Scud missile attacks were a real danger too. We got used to the sound of attack alarms and practising chemical and biological warfare drills in temperatures of 40°C and over, with full protective clothing and respirators. Diplomatic negotiations dragged on, and as December approached, with no signs of imminent combat, roulements were put in place to allow additional personnel and units to train in the environment they might be fighting in, and to give those of us sent out at no notice time to go home and recoup, on twenty-four-hours' notice to move (NTM) and return if need be. Soon after I returned home, war fighting broke out, and came to a halt again in such an unexpectedly short timescale that I played no further part. But I was happy with my contribution and preparation to fight with just minutes' notice in a country I'd never been to before.

No sooner had the Gulf War finished than 'Options for Change' began decimating the post-Cold War military. Several RAF squadrons had disbanded and competition for flying tours was high, with 75,000 jobs already cut in the RAF alone. But amidst all this, the RAF had finally opened its doors to employ female fast-jet aircrew. Many front-line aircrew welcomed the change in recruitment policy, arguing that as long as a person could do the job, then gender shouldn't be an issue ... but some seemingly took it as a personal insult and openly derided the decision! For me it was a wonderful progression and would be an important part of my life to come. If the Phantom had still been in service, my next choice of posting would have been easy. However, my draw to the RAF in the first place had been helicopters, and when my posting officer mentioned he was seeking fast-jet volunteers with air defence or 'mud-moving' experience to transfer to battlefield helicopters, I stepped up. First, I had to endure the training system once again, to learn the basics of helicopter operations. It was a nine-month course, during which one of my fellow students decided he had tolerated enough of hiding his sexuality and came out as gay. As soon as the chain of command became aware, his fate was sealed and he was dismissed from the RAF – a sad confirmation to me that the risk still existed.

In August 1993 I joined No. 60 Squadron at RAF Benson in Oxfordshire, flying the Wessex HC2. The squadron's role was to support the Army, and the

Wessex was a troop carrier. Less than two weeks after completing my Operational Conversion Course, I was flying missions in Northern Ireland, detached there to reinforce the Wessex crews on 72 Squadron, a unit that was permanently based there. The role of the British military in Northern Ireland was given the formal name 'Operation Banner' and was ordained to 'support the police and government, in allowing the population to live and work without the fear of violence and extremism'. The threat became more evident when being issued a Heckler and Koch 53 (HK 53) semi-automatic rifle and a 9mm Browning pistol to go flying in the UK! Our tasking involved moving troops and supplies in and out of Forward Operating Bases (FOBs), and inserting troops for intelligence missions, arrest operations, vehicle stop and search patrols, or 'foot patrols' along the border with Eire, by day and night. Night operations helped with covertness, but night-vision goggles were also new to me and took some getting used to. I quickly learned that the terrorists watched and adapted: if a landing point or route was used frequently it would be used for an ambush on the next visit. Unpredictability and good tactics were the key to survival, with threats including roadside bombs, heavy machine guns, small-arms fire, mortars and MANPADS (Man-Portable Air-Defence Systems) infra-red 'heat-seeking' missiles, and all but the MANPADS had been used successfully against military helicopters operating there.

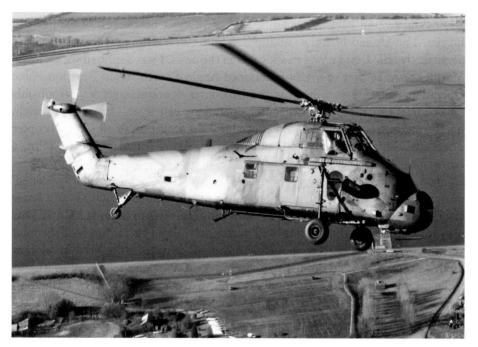

In a Wessex HC2 glinting in the sunlight, near RAF Benson, Oxfordshire, 1994.

I enjoyed the tactical flying elements and enrolled on the 1994 Helicopter Tactics Instructor Course. My professional life had direction, but I was still struggling with my personal life. As Christmas 1994 approached, I once again began questioning what life was all about. I was taking more risks to enjoy my private life as Caroline, but that wasn't enough. I wanted to be openly free of the unbearable restrictions I was placing on my life to keep my job and make everyone else happy. When I saw a magazine advert for feminising hormones my mind went wild in eager anticipation of what happiness that would bring. I invested in a supply, and on 4 January 1995, after much worrying about possible outcomes, my will finally overrode my caution and I began my treatment without any intention of declaring it to military medical staff. 'Self-medication' was against all the rules for aircrew but telling anyone at this stage meant dismissal, for sure. The results were wonderful – too wonderful in many ways – and after a couple of months, a tape measure revealed my chest size had increased by 3 inches already. I worried it was noticeable and began standing with folded arms across flying suit breast pockets 'padded' with bulgy items, taking attention away from my extra curves, as gentle as they were. I thought I would be caught out and realised I wasn't yet ready for that risk. It was a sad day when I reluctantly ceased application, but it wasn't over; I just wasn't ready yet. Then, once again, I was off to a war zone at short notice.

This time, my destination was Kiseljak, a small town of red-roofed white houses and around 7,000 inhabitants, located 18 miles north-west of Sarajevo, in Bosnia. The United Nations' attempts to end a devastating civil war there had persistently failed, and now genocide was in the news. I was deployed with a Royal Marines team as part of a UN-sanctioned Anglo-French Rapid Reaction Force Operational Staff. I was there as the helicopter operations officer, responsible for creating and running a helicopter operations cell (Heli-Ops) from scratch, for the tasking, coordination, and procedural deconfliction of all UN helicopter assets in Bosnia. I gained the company of an Army Air Corps Lynx pilot, a Norwegian Arapaho pilot, a French Puma pilot and a French warrant officer adjutant, allowing us to operate a twenty-four-hour, 7/7 watch in a 'hardened' purpose-built Tactical Air Operations and Control Centre (TAOCC) at a lower level in the building. One of my most rewarding tasks was in creating a CASEVAC plan to enable injured or critically ill personnel a rapid extraction by helicopter and delivery to the nearest appropriate trauma centre. Little did I know how often we would need to do just that, and it became especially crucial in August when a vehicle carrying the diplomatic level peace negotiation party crashed off a mountainside road near Sarajevo in a tragedy that killed many, including the American Ambassador.

On 28 August, Sarajevo market was mortared, with forty dead. Blame pointed squarely at Bosnian Serb forces, and the next day, NATO responded. Over five

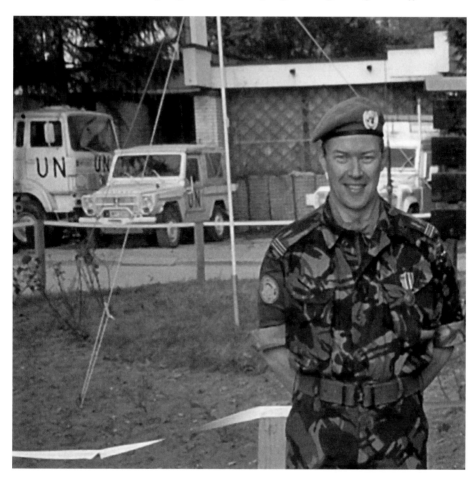

Presented with a UN Medal, and a three-month tour extension with NATO, Kiseljak, Bosnia Herzegovina, 1995.

days, aircraft and ground forces nearby engaged with Bosnian Serb Army (BSA) forces, targeting their weapons and communications. Our building was evacuated above the third floor level, so sleeping bodies cluttered the corridors of the floors below. We anticipated shelling from local BSA artillery, or attacks by enemy aircraft. A building bristling with aerials was a valid target, especially when during a planned respite, allowing the Bosnian Serb Commander time to accept terms for a more permanent cessation of hostilities, Admiral Smith appeared on CNN and stated how successful the air raids had been, and how 'It was all down to the success of the team at Kiseljak, who right now are under the noses of the BSA artillery'. We thanked him for reminding them! Finally, after a brief declaration of war on NATO, the Bosnian Serb military leader Ratko Mladić agreed to the NATO and UN demands.

NATO formally took over the mission in Bosnia, and I was 'invited' to remain behind to add my experience to their new role of implementing the peace, a mission now known as IFOR (Implementation Force), making it another three months before I got home. I had spent seven months in a war zone in a thoroughly masculine environment, and I had missed being able to be myself, in my own home. Perhaps it was the war-torn devastation I had seen around me – reinforcement that life is too short, and we should live it to our best, or at least always try – but I needed to move my own life forward now. The hormones had given me a glimpse of a better future and now I needed to do something positive about that.

In 1997, the Wessex was beginning to be removed from RAF service to make way for a new helicopter, the Merlin HC Mk3, a state-of-the-art troop carrier. I had been recommended for a job with the Rotary Wing Operational Evaluation and Training Unit (RWOETU), becoming the first aircrew posted to the RAF Merlin, and to RWOETU – a great accolade and a role I was eager to take on. My job was to liaise with the Westland factory at Yeovil, in Somerset, and the aircraft's Implementation Team, providing a military aircrew perspective and input to operating aspects of the build. With the aircraft a couple of years away from service, and the Wessex force diminishing, I was given a full conversion course on the Puma helicopter, too; little did I realise how important this would become. For now, it meant I could maintain my flying role, help with aircraft trials, teach on the tactics instructor course and still deal with Merlin introduction and operations issues. Regardless of this incredible posting, I was finally accepting that my life was mine alone to live, and that my longest held fear of losing my family was naively misplaced. I had to be true to myself, and if they loved me, they would surely support me, as hard as that may be. I set myself a series of tests, to be sure I could survive such an incredible change and to find the best way to implement it, and in the early summer of 1998, my decision was made.

***

After seeking professional private medical care through a gender psychiatrist based in London, his confirmation of gender dysphoria permitted me to resume taking hormones, but under supervision this time. I decided my best hope for telling family lay with my sister, Sandra. She lived in Morayshire, Scotland, so when tasking came in for a Puma to work with Army units for a few days near Inverness, I took the chance.

After working with troops in the Scottish Highlands, we landed at RAF Kinloss, on the southern shore of the Moray Firth, and I set off to meet Sandra at the base's main gate. She lived an hour's drive away and it was to become the longest day of my life. We sat side by side on a sofa in front of a crackling log fire, talking into the early hours, until her interest in my 'important news' reached a point where I became committed. I was scared that what I would say would lose her for ever, but once I had said a couple of vital words, there was no going back. I answered one of her questions and took the plunge, fearfully explaining how throughout all of my conscious life I had identified as female, and now I was following my heart! She had remained ever so calm, and after the briefest of pauses, took my hands in hers and replied, 'That's OK, honestly, that is OK. I love you and I was worried you were very ill. If that's all it is, there's no problem. I love you and I will be there for you ... I will help you through this.' To say it was an unbelievable and emotional moment would never do it justice. We continued talking until the sun came up, and I had a sister who now had a sister.

Next step was to tell the military, where it was still illegal to be gay and, by connection, that meant LGBT. Following the wonderful reaction of an RAF friend and his family I had confided in with the confidence of Sandra's support, we decided I should approach the RAF through the medical chain, and I needed to be sure I had all my paperwork in order as 'evidence'. Then I discovered an online story alluding to there being a sergeant major in the Army's REME who was also seeking permission to transition gender. She was called Joanne Wingate, and efforts to find more details were frustrated through confidentiality. I wasn't sure whether it was rumour or fact, but I sent her a letter through a confidential network mailing system, encouraged that there might be someone else in the military feeling the same way that I did. I needed someone else to talk to, someone who understood. Someone who was on a similar journey would be perfect, but for now I had to follow my own path.

As December 1998 approached, Joanne got in touch and we met up in London. I was delighted that she had found budding support, after a lot of effort, and was looking to transition gender in the new year, but my future remained uncertain. As much as the three services all worked to the same standards and regulations laid down by the Ministry of Defence, they all tended to 'interpret' the rules differently or provide reasons why some rules weren't appropriate for them. It could easily be argued that, due to the medical and psychological stresses involved in transitioning gender, it wasn't appropriate for me to remain as aircrew. And if I couldn't do my job, then there would be no reason for me to be retained. 'Dismissed on medical grounds' was an easy quick fix for the RAF. After what seemed an eternity of waiting, my latest gender psychiatrist's report arrived, and together with my 'information pack' of everything I could find referencing gender dysphoria, I made a double appointment to see my chosen medical officer and discover my fate. It was a day that would make or break me, but 4 February 1999 was a day that went way better than I could have ever imagined.

My explanation had grown a little emotional, but before I left Dr Katie's office, I knew I had told the right person, and that I had gained a strong ally. She cleared her desk for the remainder of the day and made phone calls, while I returned to my own work, and waited … very anxiously. An hour later, I was back in her office. Not all the phone calls had gone well; one recipient had broken her medical in confidence demands and already spread rumour, insisting I was going through a phase and would be OK after the weekend! But the most amazing news was that the decision had come down from the top, and I was to be to be allowed to transition and remain in service. It was truly wonderful, one the best of days of my life, but there was still much to do. I was the first person in the history of the RAF to do this – the first officer in the history of the British Armed Forces, even. Katie had spoken with our own station commander and reassured me he wanted to help, and he had spoken with the RAF's Personnel Management Agency to agree what happened next. We were all working without any clue of how best to handle this, but we agreed for the moment that only a small management team needed to know, until we were ready … until I was ready.

I was worried when my aircrew medical was downgraded to 'ground duties UK only' but was reassured it was only until my medical pathway was understood and complete. There was no choice, and I knew the next few months would be an emotional journey, not least because now I needed to tell my parents and brothers. I had shown them clues since that first day in Malaya, but they hadn't seen; they only saw what they wanted to see. I hoped that knowing the military was happy to retain me in service could help them understand, but I knew my family would never be the same again, and that burden was extraordinarily difficult to carry. It was Sandra who broke the news. We had agreed my being there would raise tempers, and they did flare. They couldn't believe what I was doing to them, how embarrassing it all was. My brothers broke off contact, and my relationship with my parents would never recover. Over the next couple of months, we struggled through short and difficult phone calls every couple of weeks, but they didn't want to discuss my decision. I would meet them only once as Caroline, and then never again.

The RAF agreed I should move to a new base, so I could transition with the least disturbance to my colleagues and me. It didn't feel right to expect them to cope with me turning up wearing female uniform; because this was all untrodden ground, we didn't have any real idea how it would work out. Being restricted to ground duties, it made sense to be posted to the Personnel Management Agency Headquarters at RAF Innsworth, near Gloucester. I was posted to work with Group Captain Martin Stringer, as the Ethnic Minority Recruiting Policy Team.

My first day at work was exciting, but anxious. How would people react? How would I fare? How did I look? It didn't help that my future co-workers had been briefed about my arrival and my background, destroying a key reason for me beginning my life in a new workplace. Any chance of them getting to know me without prejudging me had been lost. Now they worried about how to interact, and from my desk in the corner of a large open-plan office, I watched as twenty or so civilian and Air Force employees worked in awkward silence, making no eye contact with me. I couldn't make the first move if I was to be sure they accepted me. Eventually, one of the civilian ladies, Rose West, introduced herself and asked if I wanted to join her for a cup of tea. It was simple, but the ice was broken.

Working at Personnel Headquarters was also a perfect opportunity to help evolve the first draft of a document written to provide 'Guidance to Commanders, Supervisors and Personnel Regarding the Retention and Recruitment of Transsexual Personnel'. It was evident the MoD was committed to retaining transgender personnel, yet the ban on lesbian, gay and bisexual service personnel remained in force. Through my work with equality and policy staffs, I developed two further very close friendships – with Val Marden and Gail Kinvig, two ladies who would play an important part in building my confidence as an individual and my inclusion in things everyone else would consider routine. After a while I was sent to RAF Cranwell to work at the Department of Recruitment and Selection, known as 'Doris'. I met a young officer called Mary Jones, and she became a great mentor, especially regarding simple things, like putting my hair into a regulation 'bun', though I still preferred my hair down and long, in an attempt to hide a neck I considered ungainly (a product of twelve years of neck muscles straining to hold my head high while under high levels of G-force, during air combat in the Phantom and the Hawk).

It didn't take long before rumours began to spread. I spent some time observing an RAF recruiter's course, until one day the students all downed tools and demanded to know why there was someone in the classroom who had changed sex. 'Why was that allowed?' 'Why were they still in the military?' I was asked directly, with an angry tone, 'Why are you in my Air Force?' I was surrounded by a cacophony of demands and complaints, grievance that I was serving in the same Air Force as they were. I was shocked and disappointed. The Recruiting School commander, someone I knew from my Phantom days at RAF Leuchars, was appalled with their reactions, and questioned their own fitness to serve in Careers Offices with such attitudes. A vocal minority had triggered shock and confusion by revealing something without all the facts. They made everyone else believe it was wrong and unlawful to 'have a transsexual in the military'. To a degree, I could see why that argument would be offered with LGB service still not permitted, and people wrongly assuming that being 'transsexual' was a matter of sexual identity. The outspoken students in the room were quick to back down when they realised their careers were now more questionable than mine was, but I had now seen evidence that my acceptance wasn't going to be straightforward within the wider military.

I was still keen to return to flying duties, but my temporary employment was invaluable in giving me and the RAF time to adjust. We were all learning from the good and not so good experiences, and what we were learning would help others

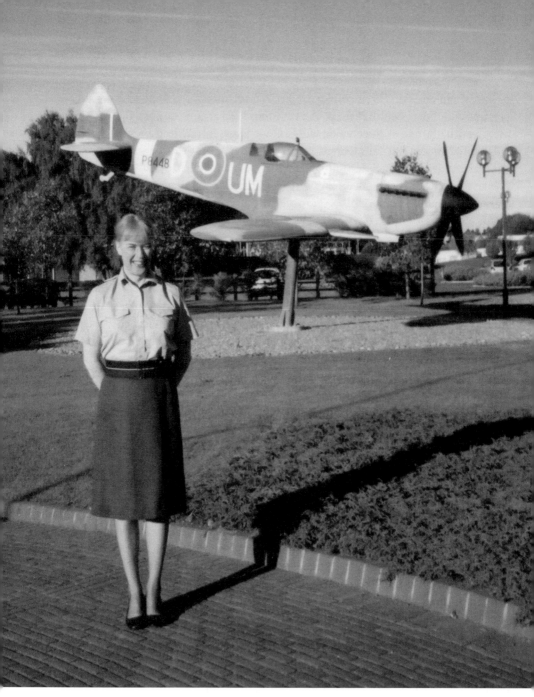

A year post-transition, so much happier, but my challenges were just beginning. RAF Cranwell, 2000.

in the future. When the senior officer commanding Supply sent out an email, copying in many people who had no right to know, stating, 'Flight Lieutenant Paige will be visiting Clothing Stores tomorrow at 10 a.m. He is to be issued female uniform in accordance with the following list, in replacement to his male uniform,' he earned a swift rebuke from my boss, and uniform issue procedures in the 'policy' guidance document were amended.

On 12 January 2000, the Ministry of Defence was finally made to repeal its law against gay military service, and LGB personnel were able to serve openly. But the military system still wasn't ready for that: decades of structured condemnation and hostility couldn't be transformed overnight, and it remained a scary and sceptical place in which to come out. Then, in August 2000, I was summoned to my boss's office. *The Sun* newspaper had my details and was going to print an article. From what they had told the Ministry of Defence, the only information they had correct was my name. I had been a serving female officer for sixteen months without any press attention, and it had lulled me into a false sense of security, neglecting the ever-present risk of public exposure, and worse, public exposure of a secret that my family had kept from the rest of their family, friends and neighbours. I asked for an opportunity to turn the story around and make it factual, and the MoD and newspaper agreed to an interview at MoD Main Building in London. After John Kay, *The Sun*'s chief reporter, seemed to warm to my account, he switched tack to a personal interest story instead of the expected mocking one. The result was a front-page headline five days later, and then my world started crashing around me. Fortunately, I had the support of my friends at RAF Innsworth, but what happened next gave me doubt I would be able to return to flying duties and triggered a family split, my longest held fear.

The paternal side of my family expressed open hostility towards me, but my maternal aunties, uncles and cousins only expressed love and support. Newspapers, including *The Sun*, began running articles and reactions that introduced 'experts' from unqualified sources. A retired Army colonel questioned my retention in the military, insisting that people like me 'would be a liability on operations, and couldn't be issued a weapon, because I clearly had a mental health problem'. And if I couldn't bear a weapon, I 'had no place in the military'. I had already served in war zones, concealing my inner struggles, yet I had never allowed it to affect my expected performance, which surely demonstrated a tremendously resilient mental health. And free of my distress, if anything, my focus was 100 per cent now, not having to worry about a disciplinary hearing, followed by humiliation and dismissal from my job. And I had certificates of being mentally healthy from three independent psychiatrists, two of them gender specialists, and one a military specialist. But then others joined in, an online forum for aircrew added similar disgust and reasoning, and feeling was turning rapidly against my continued service. People who didn't understand became instant experts, joining in, all voicing opinions on why a 'transsexual' person had no place in today's military. I was truly seeing what people thought of me, publicly and from within the military too, and it looked like a flying unit was going to become an unwelcoming place to be. It was demoralising, and I feared for my future on the front line. Then, finally, I began to see hope. After a week that had seemingly stretched to eternity, opinions began to transform: positive comments were being expressed, referring to my professional ability, or positive experiences individuals had shared with me, arguing that doing the job was all that mattered. The negative opinions were still there, but they were becoming overwhelmed. It had taken just one military voice to stand up for me, and the rest followed. Perhaps being seen standing up for something so 'controversial' had caused reluctance to be first, but each voice that now followed inspired me more, and it was time to find out if I did have a future back on a squadron.

***

Of the several options my desk officer offered, I only wanted one: the Merlin HC Mk3. It would be coming into service in the next year and I was keen to be reacquainted. As a tactical battlefield helicopter, Merlin would also give me the opportunity to prove these voices wrong, to show that I could serve on the front line, that being transgender was of no consequence. Of the 2 per cent female of 4,246 aircrew in the RAF, I was the only one who was transgender; I knew it was going to be my biggest challenge yet. At 8.55 am on Monday, 4 December 2000, I arrived at the squadron, in the very same hangar I had worked in before I changed my life around. In the squadron's crew room I met five aircrew with whom I was going to be working closely, and after a brief awkward 'how do we start inclusive conversation here', the ice was broken and we began what would become great friendships.

The troop-carrying version of the Merlin was not due to begin arriving into RAF service until March 2001, and the squadron's reformation deadline was a royal parade and celebration just seven months away. My role was to become the squadron helicopter tactics instructor, and I needed to learn the aircraft systems to do this; the Merlin was coming into service with one of the most technologically advanced defensive aids systems in the world. I decided to use my time learning and relearning as much about tactics, electronic warfare and defensive systems as I could. In the space of three months I had been on three major courses, plus two tactics conferences at the Air Warfare Centre at RAF Waddington in Lincolnshire, and I had gained a higher security clearance to help. I was the first transgender person to be posted to a front-line unit in any of the Armed Forces and I couldn't afford to fail. Joanne hadn't been allowed to return to her unit and was approaching her regular army service leaving point. She couldn't stay longer but she could be proud of her work with transgender policy guidance, ensuring others in the future would be far better supported.

But life wasn't easy, and no LGBT support network yet existed in the military. It is one thing being authorised to stay in service; it's another working in an environment that doesn't want you there. Hostility was just around the corner and several people of all ranks, including former very close friends from my Phantom days, made it expressly clear that I wasn't wanted. Fortunately, I had also reacquainted with friends who added positivity to my life.

On 1 July 2001, No. 28 (Army Cooperation) Squadron officially reformed, with Prince Michael of Kent taking the salute. On 9 September, I was at RAF Mildenhall briefing the US 21st Special Operations Squadron's (SOS) MH-53 aircrew on the Merlin's capabilities, when we saw on an ops room TV horrific images of aircraft hitting New York's World Trade Center ... and the world changed for the worse.

Thankfully, I had recently passed my medical board, and a year after the squadron's reformation, I began the No. 1 Merlin Operational Conversion Course. After completing that we began working the aircraft up for operational clearances. But then life took a downward turn. Being a transgender woman in a goldfish bowl still wasn't easy; opportunistic harassment was never far away, and flying and learning a complicated aircraft was extremely demanding. I was working hard but not getting the results I wanted in the cockpit. The boss failed me on a 'Combat Ready' qualification, and then my dad died – a heart attack. I was angry when my 'family' barred me from attending his funeral, but I was tormented, too, that we had lost for ever any opportunity for reconciliation. On top of this, my relationship with squadron friends had grown strained, and I was having doubts in my own abilities.

The boss sent me to see the Medical Officer, worried for my mental health, but if I was signed off as unfit now, I saw no way back to flying duties. Fortunately, she determined I was doing my best in extraordinary circumstances but was still fit to fly. I was given an opportunity to slow down the pace a little, and it paid off when I achieved an excellent result on my next 'Combat Ready' check. My confidence was restored, but I knew I still had a long way to go, a lot to prove. Then war came, again. Merlin was still not fully operational, so we weren't able to join our sister units in Iraq in 2003, but we went to Bosnia instead, to continue building our experience with the aircraft in testing environments, supporting NATO's Stability Augmentation Forces and hunting PIFWCs (persons indicted for war crimes).

In August 2004, it was announced our squadron would be deploying to southern Iraq in the new year in support of Operation Telic, providing support to coalition and Iraqi troops. I was disappointed when I wasn't included amongst the first crews selected to go. I had worked hard to be the lead squadron tactics instructor, and I knew the protection systems fitted to our aircraft better than anyone else, a responsibility I took seriously. I had been visiting the Air Warfare Centre to keep abreast of tactical matters and threat capabilities, but during one visit I was shown some unsettling news. An essential part of an onboard system wasn't working as it was meant to, making the aircraft unsafe to deploy to a high threat environment.

I had a responsibility to make sure the crews were as well prepared as they could be, to help minimise any risk for operating Merlin in such a hostile theatre, but my commanders failed to accept my concerns. I invited the experts down to give the crews a briefing, then they listened, and we identified a solution. Now I was rewarded with inclusion on the first detachment of Merlin going to Iraq. My place was on the first detachment, not the second or third: I had to experience the environment first-hand as soon as possible, if I was going to learn and teach how to better survive there. Inclusion was the key to me for many reasons, but my determination and knowledge would prove essential on detachments yet to come.

We had four aircraft in theatre, with four full crews and a detachment commander. Merlin was replacing Chinook, and rumour control had said it wasn't good enough. Our first challenge was to prove this wrong, and we did so by exceeding every test put before us. Merlin also brought an advantage of range, one that was to prove valuable in reaching insurgents who crossed previously unpatrolled borders, and for reaching critically injured or seriously ill ground forces with an onboard medical team, before extracting them to the nearest trauma centre for critical care, a casualty evacuation role known in theatre as Medical Immediate Response Team (MIRT). It would prove to be one of our most demanding and dangerous, but most rewarding roles.

General tasking out of Basra included moving troops and supplies in and out of forward operating bases, inserting troops for counter-insurgency operations and

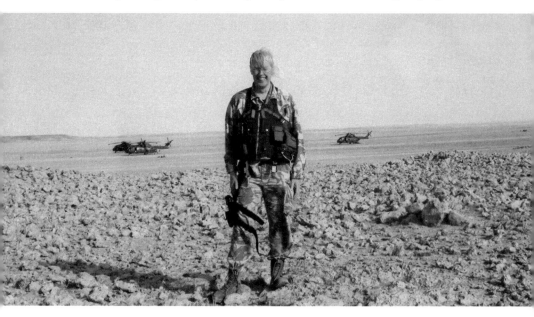

Deep into the Al Muthanna Desert, Iraq, 2005, awaiting a 'Go' during a three-ship long range interdiction mission.

extracting them when need be, vehicle stop and search patrols, recce tasks, and convoy escort, all by day or night. We also provided an Airborne Reaction Force (ARF) with troops, on standby with us, or an Explosives Ordnance Team (EOD), or a MIRT. A crew and aircraft rotated for two days at a time to Al Amarah, an hour's flight time to the north, or Camp Smyth VC, seventy minutes' flight to the west, primarily for MIRT but also ARF. Al Amarah was regularly rocketed, and the first time I experienced this, the rockets hit a perimeter wall surrounding our aircraft, narrowly missing our adjacent crew room and an EOD team resting nearby. Immediately after the explosion, everything went eerily quiet and we looked at each other questioningly, until the shriek of the mortar alarm settled any doubt. While everyone else sought shelter, we scrambled to our aircraft, *Foxy*, expecting an ARF to join us, but although the aircraft initially failed to start and we waited as long as we dare, we were airborne without any sight of them. The aircraft was better off in the air, able to react to casualty evacuation or spot and track the firing team.

After my first Iraq tour I was posted back to RWOETU, the very unit I had been on when I made my decision to live my life openly, back in 1998. Being on the squadron meant a lot to me, but it also made sense to be part of RWOETU, with the knowledge, skills and current operational experience I had gained. There was much to be done to help evolve the protection of aircraft flying in war zones, and I wanted to be part of that. RWOETU was responsible for evaluating everything from operating software and control systems to personal equipment, with added responsibility to develop procedures, guidance and training for squadron crews. I was still declared part of the squadron's Combat Ready allocation, so I needed to keep my skill levels and knowledge to the highest of standards, more so because now I was looked upon by the squadron as an expert on all matters. RWOETU's Merlin desk was a team of three, and my speciality

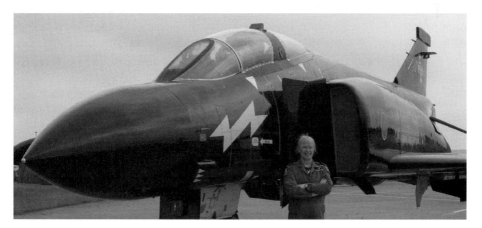

Reunited with F4 Phantom *Black Mike* during a Helicopter Tactics Instructor course, RAF Leuchars, 2006.

became tactics, electronic warfare and platform protection. Once a year, we also helped instruct trainee tactics instructors on the seven-week Helicopter Tactics Instructor Course, including RAF, Army Air Corps (AAC) and RN Commando Helicopter Force (CHF) trainees – a course I had been instructing on annually since my own qualification in 1994.

Then, on Saturday, 6 May 2006, a Lynx helicopter was hit by a MANPADS missile over Basra city, exploding and killing all five people on board. Along with the three-man crew were two people I knew very well and counted as good friends, John Coxen, my boss at RWOETU, and Sarah Mulvihill, the squadron's Operations Officer. It was a cruel reminder of how dangerous those skies were, and why it was vital to get my job right.

Six months later, I deployed to Iraq for the second time. This time I was delighted to be crewed with Kat England for the first half of my tour, and Michelle Goodman for the second half, a female front-end aircraft. Basra airfield was being rocketed now, too, at least once a day, often twice or more, but something else would focus my expertise – this time, the consequences of a fatal explosion in England, in a factory responsible for supplying a critical part of our defensive systems, our infrared decoy flares. When orders came down to switch our flare systems to manual, the risk of losing an aircraft due to a missile engagement went up, considerably. The order was intended to prevent flares being released on a false alarm, but it also took away protection on a real alarm. In automatic mode, the system would take no chances: if it thought it had detected a missile threat, it would trigger countermeasures immediately. Split seconds in reaction time meant the difference between life or death for up to twenty-eight people on each Merlin. In manual mode our system only provided detection and warning, relying on the crew to then initiate flare release, but by the time they could process and react, it would already be too late. When we became the first crew ordered to fly with manual settings, I advised otherwise. I wasn't in the habit of ignoring orders, but this was my job and speciality, and after landing from the mission I explained my concerns to the boss. He asked if I had a solution, and I did, but it was unconventional and would need consideration and approval from specialist agencies in the UK. Within hours we had received a yes. We could reduce the amount of flare usage, but without reducing the aircraft's protection. It meant we could still fly in 'auto', but it required software changes to systems that would usually take several weeks to process and authorise. The team in the UK worked wonders; within three days we had the new data and I briefed the crews on the new procedures. It carried us through until the supply chain was restored, so everyone was happy, and I had directly influenced the continued operational readiness and safety of Merlin missions in Iraq. I also gained tremendous respect from my colleagues, knowing I had their backs, as they had mine. Seven years had passed since critics of my military service had voiced their opinions to the press, that I would be a liability on operations, a danger to colleagues, and now their arguments were once again proven as malicious presumptions.

In 2007, I was summoned to my flight commander's office to be greeted with a handshake and news that Commander Joint Helicopter Command (JHC) was awarding me his commendation 'for the exceptional work you have done regarding Merlin's defensive aids and your efforts out in Iraq'. I appreciated that he would have written me up for that, but the fact that a two-star Army general had put his name to it was incredibly uplifting. Yet despite all my efforts and achievements in Iraq, away from the company of my colleagues and friends I was still being harassed, for being transgender. Even though we were all risking our lives together in facing a common threat, I still couldn't go to the gym or dining tent without people staring, gossiping and sniggering. Women made up less than 9 per cent of the forces, as an average, and we all had to put up with staring from males, but I knew the attention directed at me wasn't one of 'eye candy'. It was puzzlement, reservation and sometimes, unsubtle disrespect. Comments grew louder as I passed by groups, making sure I knew they knew my background; ugly comments and laughs about me, not with me. I was never aware of anyone intervening; although I suspected the majority of personnel shared impartial or even positive opinions about my standing on the line with them, they remained silent. The negative comments weren't being balanced out or redressed, and so they hit harder. It wasn't just banter, either. Banter is important to the military, and I would never wish to restrict it, but there's a fine line between banter and intimidation, and some people didn't know the boundaries. Those who knew me, or of my military experience and skills, offered friendship, respect or support; those who didn't know me were vulnerable to negative judgements based on rumour, misinformation or bigoted opinions. I realised education was the key to understanding, and understanding was the key to respect, so on my return to the UK, I contacted the boss of the tri-service Diversity and Inclusion Training School at RAF Shrivenham, Michelle Randall, and volunteered time to help raise awareness on what it actually meant to be transgender. And I gained another great friendship on the way. Michelle had organised a Diversity and Inclusion Roadshow and invited me to join it, visiting RAF bases and speaking of my experiences to personnel managers, medical professionals and various other listeners. It ended with me speaking at the first tri-service Diversity Conference, in London. I was still advising on current and future policy, for all three services, and also as an active member of the RAF LGBT Forum, combining invaluable experiences, advice, guidance and motivation to improve the inclusion of all LGBT personnel in the British Armed Forces. Inclusion was significantly better than it had ever been, but my experiences in Iraq were evidence there was still much to do.

I completed two more tours in Iraq, and each had occasions where my knowledge, experience and skill contributed to the safe flight of not just Merlin

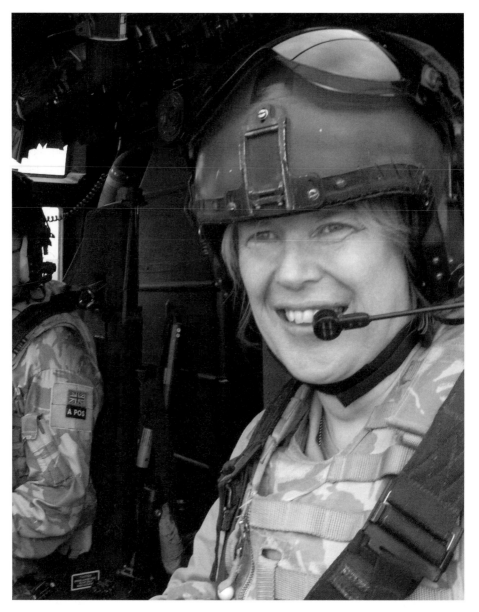

On task in 'my office', the cockpit of a Merlin HC Mk3, somewhere in Iraq, 2009.

helicopters, but other aircraft including large transport aircraft, UK and US. In 2009, with the UK's involvement in Iraq winding down, Merlin was earmarked to join with the Chinooks operating in Helmand Province, Afghanistan. I was determined to go with the first deployment for all the same reasons I'd pushed hard to go to Iraq. It was a new mission, with a new enemy, for Merlin at least, and that meant different threats and enemy tactics. History had taught the world never to underestimate the low-tech adversary that existed in Afghanistan. The Soviet Union had lost over 300 helicopters there in nine years following their invasion in 1979. It was an extremely dangerous part of the world to fly in. We had gained new defensive systems following evaluations we had flown in the deserts of Iraq in 2008, but the chalk-like dust in Afghanistan meant the aircraft, equipment and people would need additional safeguards and procedures. When I identified issues with the placement and lack of associated crew warning regarding critical 'safety switches' in the cockpit, I needed to prove the risk before people would spend any time and money on fixing it, so I did, and presented a solution that could be incorporated with concurrent upgrades. I was delighted when I first saw the new system in place and preventing a crew from a potentially disastrous mistake, with the reassuringly straightforward way the crew used it – further evidence that I was making a difference.

***

Afghanistan required a very different way of operating compared to Iraq, and that made it more important for me that I was there. There had been a lot of investment, and for good reason: a UK casualty list already numbered hundreds killed. Landing sites had diverse threat levels and, depending on the level of risk, required a minimum of two helicopters supporting each other, or at least one Lynx as escort, or a pair of Apaches in escort for the highest risk tasking, if they were available. My first two deployments to Camp Bastion in Afghanistan were to focus on the evaluation of platform protection systems, and what we learned had invaluable benefit for other platforms, US and UK, but I was also keen to ensure the tactics were right and used properly. There were an awful lot of people on the ground reaching into cockpits and enforcing actions from the detached safety of their desk. I needed to make sure crews had the best information available to make the most appropriate decision, and to stand up against obstinacy. There was much to lose.

My determination was working, and in 2010 I received a second commendation 'for exceptional service', this time from a rear admiral. The citation read: 'for dedication, drive and real desire to ensure the Merlin Force aircraft and crews were protected as best as possible', for being a 'significant driving force, operating at a level normally expected of individuals of considerably higher rank', for 'enabling the delivery of operational capability', and for 'single-handedly writing tactical advice and crew training, whilst standing firm against intransigence and operational pressure to ensure the best possible protection'.

In September 2011, my desk officer decided it was time for me to move from RWOETU. I only had three years left before I reached my maximum age for

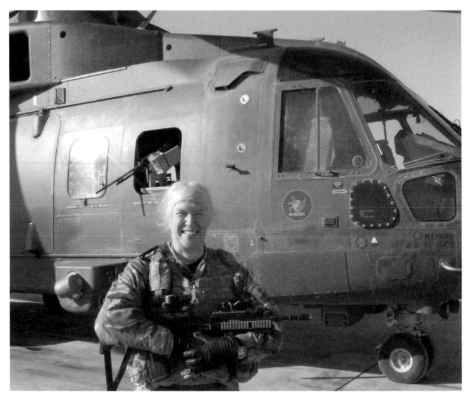

Post-mission photo during my final operational tour, Camp Bastion, Afghanistan, 2013.

service, and could easily have asked for a 'restful job', ready for retirement. However, I didn't want to just drop my experience and knowledge when my colleagues and friends were still in Afghanistan, and I wanted to end my flying career from a front-line role, so I asked to go back to No. 28 (AC) Squadron, from where I had seen Merlin into service.

On New Year's Eve, during my third time in Afghanistan, my flight commander approached and said, 'Caz, as it is near midnight, I can now tell you that you have been awarded a Commander-in-Chief Air Command Commendation in the Queen's New Year's Honours List.' I didn't know what to say, and what a place to be told! My third commendation 'for exceptional service' came from an RAF air marshal and, together with a 'People's Award' in 2011 from the Permanent Under-Secretary for Defence ('for trailblazing transgender service and being an outstanding role model in the UK Armed Forces'), added to the evidence that transgender people weren't any kind of risk to operational service, that given the chance, their skills and experience were as valuable and focused as any service member's.

UK forces and Merlin were soon to be pulling out of Afghanistan and my 2012/13 tour was to be my last. It seemed somewhat ironic that of all the times

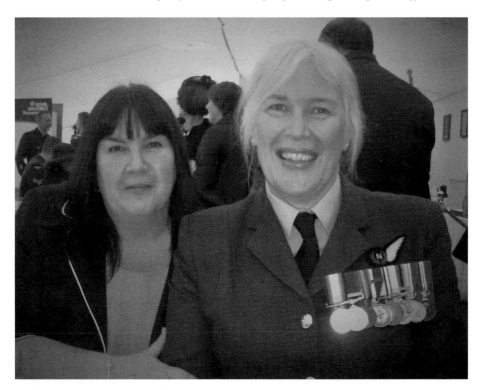

With my sister, Sandra, at the Queen's Diamond Jubilee Muster of Troops, Windsor Castle, 2012, invited in recognition of my 2012 Queen's New Year's Honours List award.

that bullets, rockets and more had passed or landed uncomfortably close to me, it would be on this final tour of duty that our aircraft was hit, causing us to divert into Lashkar Gar leaking fuel, fortunately with no casualties.

***

Back at Benson, everything was changing. A political deal meant Merlin was going to the Navy, and as Navy crews and engineers began arriving at RAF Benson, the flying became focused on their training and my job was winding down. The UK had been approached by the European Defence Agency (EDA) because they liked what they saw of the way Joint Helicopter Command trained its battlefield helicopter crews tactically. Mike Gallagher, a Puma navigator and friend I had worked with previously on RWOETU, was now running the Tactics and Training Flight, and became responsible for developing, organising and managing a European version of our own Helicopter Tactics Instructor Course (HTIC). It was a huge task, so he negotiated my loan from 28 Squadron to help. In April 2013, the EDA's No. 1 HTIC met at RAF Linton-on-Ouse, near York, for three weeks of ground

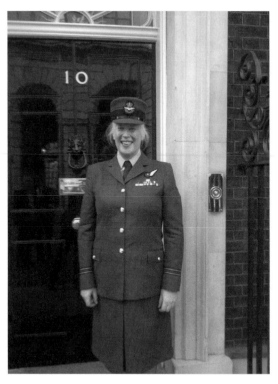

At a Prime Minister's reception for inspirational LGBT champions, 10 Downing Street, London, 2013.

instruction and simulator work, and then reconvened at Vidsel, in northern Sweden, for a three-week flying phase to put it all into practice. We had a mix of aircraft, from the venerable UH-1 'Huey' to the giant CH-53. Crews and aircraft came from Austria, Belgium, Germany and Sweden, and observers from Estonia, Hungary and Portugal. I was paired with a German 'Huey' crew, and my primary student, a confident German pilot called Till, took the 'Top Student' prize, and we became good friends. I evidently made a good impression with the European crews and I now enjoyed a multinational group of friends. Nobody questioned my suitability to be doing the job, though Till told me one evening, 'Yes, I guessed your secret the first time we met.' That was all he ever said about it, after a few drinks. It never became an issue. I always believed my circumstances were glaringly obvious, especially the minute I started talking, but I had found respect and acceptance amongst an international group, and it was really nice. Especially when on the following year's course, my primary student, a Czech Mi 171 'Hip' pilot, also took the 'Top Student' award. But the best of this was that I felt I had become an ambassador for military transgender service amongst these nations, and including the US military, and beyond. I hoped this would make a difference but at the very least, there were a growing number of people who saw the skills that would have been lost had I been dismissed when I revealed my gender identity.

As I approached my retirement point, I knew now was a good time to hang up my wings and finish my flying career – and what a career I had been fortunate enough to enjoy: over 5,000 hours of military flying in thirty-five years, crewing, instructing or evaluating in twenty-two different aircraft types, experiencing over a dozen more, and completing eighteen operational tours. And I had come to enjoy the most amazing sixteen of those years as Caroline – a journey I had never expected the day I 'signed on the dotted line'. On my fifty-fifth birthday, I walked onto a base I had served at since 1993, apart from a short break to transition, and handed in all the last pieces of my military identity. I bade a few sad goodbyes, but there was no ceremony or formal farewell. I spoke to my squadron commander for the last time, and that was it. I was a veteran.

But my military journey didn't end there. A year later, I was invited back to work alongside an EDA-contracted team, to continue teaching helicopter tactics to European military crews, this time as a civilian contractor; it was an offer I just couldn't refuse. Mike Gallagher was still the chief instructor responsible for managing and developing the courses and now I would help him do that. The course still had interest from the UK, too, with instructors and trainees. Previously I had worried some nations might find it difficult receiving instruction from a transgender woman; now it was whether they would accept instruction from a civilian. But once again, it was needless apprehension. I was a veteran, not a civilian, with a lot of experience and knowledge to share, and that is where their respect lay. I was delighted that my extensive experience was not just fading into the past, that I could share the matters I enjoyed teaching, and that I could still contribute to the safety of not just UK crews on operations, but of European crews and assets too. It was a wonderful gift to be able to share. And one that I still share to this day.

With Olivia Beattie at Biteback Publishing, London, 2017. Publishing day for my autobiography, *True Colours* – helping to raise awareness of transgender lives, in addition to my public speaking and media interviews.

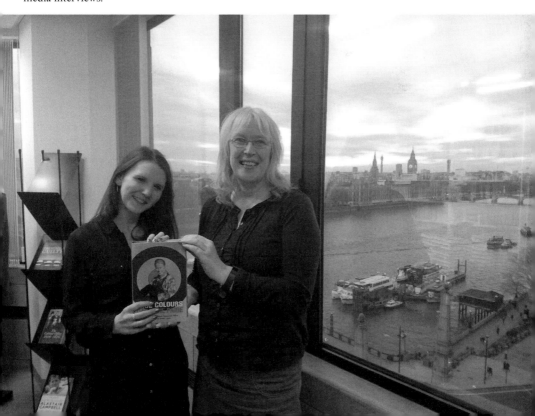

Chapter 6

Redcap Revealed
Sergeant Darren Ford
Royal Military Police

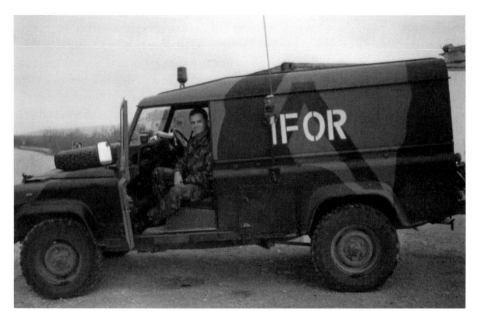

Sergeant Darren Ford, working with the NATO Implementation Force (IFOR), Tomislavgrad, Bosnia.

I was about 11 years old when I came to realise that I was different. At first it was an inkling, as I looked around and all my mates were fancying girls. But my curiosity rested with my mates and I'm sure my eyes must have betrayed me once or twice. With the benefit of hindsight, my sexuality has never really changed through my life, but we find ourselves from time to time in places and amongst people that lead us against the tide. There's certainly been quite a bit of that in my life.

My family life at the time was never great. We were a large family squashed into a small three-bedroomed house and I could not wait to get out, but that wasn't really what led me to the Army. My uncle sort of 'ran' the housing estate where he and his family lived, and our household never seemed to be without the latest

VHS video recorder, games console, microwave or other electrical goods. Dodgy? Maybe not all of it. But despite coming from an extended family, which was well known to Merseyside Police for all the wrong reasons, what I really wanted was to be a police officer. That's me swimming against the tide again. So, having almost completed sixth form at school, proud of my many O and A levels and with my nineteenth birthday looming, I applied to Merseyside Police. I'm convinced that the guy who interviewed me must have laughed his ass off as I left the room. I had seen nothing of the world, obviously. I was a little shy and wearing my dad's best jacket, which was three sizes too big and probably dodgy as well. At least I had checked that the price tag wasn't still stuck to it somewhere. The interview didn't go well, and the guy didn't even say 'Come back in a few years, son'. Unsure of which way to turn, I again met with the careers officer at school and he suggested the Army's Royal Military Police. Yeah, well, I'd never heard of them and my first instinct was that it might involve spending a lot of time trudging through mud in the pouring rain, but along I went to the Armed Forces Careers Office in Liverpool. I said nothing to my family about what I wanted to do policewise as that just wouldn't have gone down too well. The initial interview and appraisal went well and they agreed to send me to an assessment weekend within a month for formal evaluation. I felt it was right to tell my family and I started the conversation by telling Mum and Dad that I was joining the Army. A wave of pride spread across our lounge and I could sense their contentment. Then I said it was the Royal Military Police, and bugger me if that tide didn't turn back again!

The closer I got to the assessment weekend, the more I became aware of the role of the RMP and also of the operations that the Army was involved with. At the time, the Cold War was very real and tens of thousands of troops were in Germany. Northern Ireland was experiencing one of its most bloody periods and it was not so many years following the Falklands War. I would be joining an army that had very real and very important work to do and I became increasingly excited by the opportunity to do something with my life that would be important. I began to feel that I had found a purpose.

So off I went for assessment, where there were about 100 guys aged somewhere between 16 and 21. We were there for the weekend and the candidates were applying to be in just about every corps or regiment in the Army. This was the first time I began to realise that the Redcaps (Royal Military Police) were different. It's where I first heard the banter, which sets them apart, through necessity, from their Army peers.

I can still clearly remember us all sitting on the floor and being briefed about what was going to happen that weekend, especially when one of the NCOs asked, 'Who's going into the military police?' Of course, a small number of hands went up. 'Yeah? Well stand up! Right, everyone else, look around; these arseholes are going to be arresting you in a year's time.' I confess a cheeky grin crept onto my face, though I do also remember thinking, 'Oh God, what have I got myself into? One of these days I'll swim with the tide.' Even on reflection I would say that I was not obviously gay (to an outsider, anyway).

On the Saturday evening of the assessment weekend the time came around for food in the mess hall, and showers. 'Showers. Oh shit.' It would be the first time I'd seen that many guys of my age or older entirely naked, and I was suddenly paralysed with fear of being quite literally 'boned out', but I got through by keeping my eyes firmly fixed on the floor! That night a few of the candidates settled early and we were all horsing around, up and down the corridors. For many they were away from home for the first time. Earlier in the day I'd been sat with a guy who was hoping to join the 2nd Battalion The Mercian Regiment. He was friendly and somehow we caught each other's eye. Perhaps it was the beginnings of my gaydar. We chatted for a bit and then he went off to join a group of lads who were running up and down the corridors generally causing mayhem. It wasn't my thing to get involved in all that and besides, wasn't I joining the Redcaps? I was supposed to stand back from that and turn in, set an example, right?

The light in my room was off, but the space was dimly lit through the open door. No chance of sleep anytime soon with the crazies running around. The Mercian suddenly burst into the room, howling like a banshee, and jumped all over me in his boxers. Obviously I couldn't show any sign of weakness so I wrestled him as we both laughed until we fell off the bed to the floor with a thump, with him straddling me, holding my arms down. The laughing quickly turned to silence as we both just looked at each other, time freezing momentarily as he pressed himself into me, his hips barely moving, but deliberately … just enough. Growing excitement and sudden realisation made time click back to normal and we both sort of chuckled as he got from on top of me … but there was a 'moment' of tenderness, raw wanting and unspoken understanding.

Somehow it made me think that perhaps there could be a balance of life in the Army for me and that the complexities of being a gay soldier might not be quite as much of a conflict as I had imagined, and certainly not how my life had been thus far. Growing up, I'd been acutely aware that my family were of the view that all gays should be rounded up in a field and shot (that's softened a bit now!). It was never in my nature to fly a rainbow flag and it's still not today – so maybe it would work out. I knew I'd have to tread very carefully, though, whatever I did. I knew I couldn't trust anyone with my secret.

So I eventually joined in September 1986, excited to leave home and with one month of basic training at RMP Chichester followed by five months of military and civil law. I absolutely loved and hated it at the same time. We were constantly tested, continually pushed to our limits and always expected to shrug off the pain, anger or frustration. None of us realised at the time why it was so demanding but they were training us to be independent and self-sufficient to the extent where, as future Military Policemen (MPs), we could think quickly on our feet and deal with almost anything. Being thrown in with a platoon full of southerners and their different accents was fantastic as it was also something new. With each week that passed, my Scouse accent moved a few miles further south. I made some decent friends during training and, in honesty, I fancied quite a few of them, but I kept that to myself and mainly concentrated on being the best soldier I could be.

There's a lot of horseplay and banter in the Army and I know it's the same in the Air Force and the Navy. Bring together young lads in their teens and early twenties, in very close proximity where they all get to know each other incredibly well, add to the mix a generous sprinkling of alcohol and camaraderie, and it is guaranteed to bring its own brand of fun. Some of the horsing around had a quite a strong sexual tone and it was intimate in a way, but not gay; just young lads having a good time. Even during basic training, the Royal Military Police were completely segregated in that we had our own barracks, canteens and mess, bar and everything. That's another reason why I didn't meet a like-minded soldier from another cap badge in training, but it didn't matter; I was having the time of my life, doing something I felt proud of, feeling accomplished each week and with a brilliant future ahead of me.

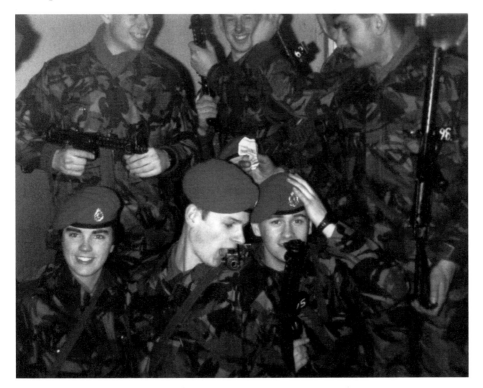

Royal Military Police Training Centre, Chichester, 1986, deploying a particularly well-shaped beret, which I quickly became very proud of.

Our training was soon coming to a close and after starting with a squad of around seventy young lads just six months earlier, we had been whittled down to around twenty-five, with our future postings about to be announced. I couldn't believe my luck. I was being posted to 2RMP in West Berlin, the largest and most prestigious RMP unit. It was 1987, and the wall stood strong and testament to the foolishness of the Cold War. But the writing was on the wall and even on arrival, I sensed change. This unit had a variety of duties to perform, including the processing of British service personnel who had asked to visit East Berlin at the world-renowned Checkpoint Charlie. At the outset I knew it would be exciting work and I couldn't wait to get started.

As the intensity of my training abated and I had time to reflect, I became more aware of the risk that being gay posed on my career and my future. There was nothing for me jobwise in Merseyside. I had left my childhood and family life behind, and the prospect of being on the dole frightened me. There was so much for me in the Army; I had found my home. Being found out to be gay wasn't just a case of being booted out. There would be no 'Red Book' (service record), there would be no pension, no support, and you might well have ended up in military prison.

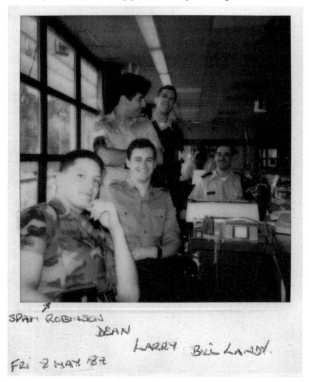

SPAN ROBINSON
DEAN
LARRY BILL LANDY.
FRI 8 MAY '87

Working with our American counterparts at Checkpoint Bravo to process service personnel leaving West Berlin, 1988.

Homosexuality was still illegal for members of the Armed Forces until the year 2000. In all transgressions of military law, the RMP were treated harshly: they knew better, and courts martial also knew that.

Nevertheless, my first gay experience was in Berlin. I dated a German girl for a couple of years, meeting her soon after I arrived in the unit. Dating girls was the norm and I did feel a need to fit in. But I also gradually and steadily became very friendly with a fellow MP. He was older than me and there was a brotherly feel to our friendship. But our friendship didn't go further than sitting next to each other and leaning on each other. I was nervous; there was a lot to lose, but from the outset I welcomed this scrap of intimacy.

There were around 100 RMPs in my unit. It was probably the largest operational police unit in the Army at the time, reflecting the importance of our work at the famous Checkpoint Charlie wall patrols and, of course, not forgetting Checkpoint Bravo, which led to the narrow vehicle corridor through East to West Germany. We also conducted patrols in the city and I preferred that work far more, because you got out and about meeting people, investigating crimes and, of a night shift, looking for underaged squaddies drinking in bars, which they were banned from until they were 18.

The wall patrol had enjoyable moments, that's for sure. I can still clearly remember standing atop of the Reichstag, throwing stones at the East Berlin border guards. Hey, we were still human and had to entertain ourselves. Being on wall patrol meant escorting twenty Soviet soldiers from one of the border crossings to Tiergarten Police Post, adjacent to the Soviet war memorial, each morning. Around 2.00 am, we would try to get our heads down for a few hours, but I'm convinced the Soviet intelligence officer knew this and took great delight in pressing the buzzer from their compound to get us out and speak with us. Didn't speak English? Yeah, OK. We used to get some good exchanges, though, with cap badges, uniform etc. Perhaps the saddest part of my role was seeing ordinary Germans from East and West Berlin who were separated from their families and

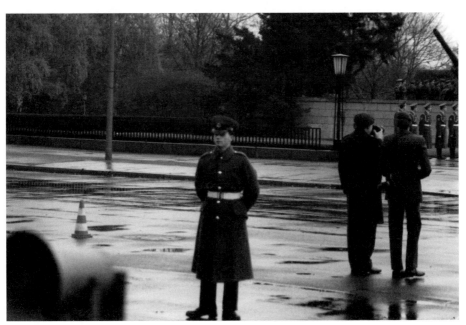

On ceremonial duties at the Soviet War Memorial, West Berlin, 1987.

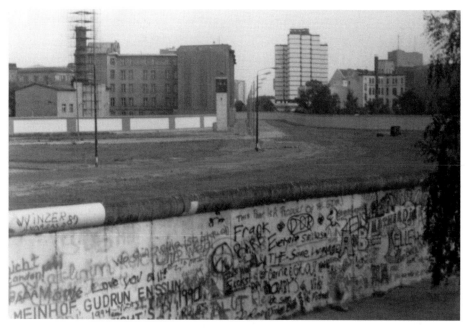

West to East. Looking across the Berlin Wall to East Berlin, 1988.

friends, trudging across the border, on one side blessed with everything that the West had to offer, and on the East side, beset with the privations of the Soviet block at that time. You could see the weariness and desperation in their faces as they came from the East in the morning and trudged back in the evening. At least those who were allowed daily transit visas got to see what they might hope for in the future.

Throughout the year, at sporadic intervals there would be an exercise known as 'Rocking Horse', which was later changed to 'Bear Defender'. There was never any warning for this exercise, which was designed to test response times of our forces if Soviet tanks started rolling into West Berlin. 2RMP were always one of the first units to have the alarm triggered by its ear-splitting siren, and we all knew what it meant. It's quite a sight to see 100 MPs knowing exactly what they had to do, where to go etc. If you were lucky enough, you would already be on night patrol and quickly divert with blue light and siren to key married quarter areas to announce 'Exercise, exercise, exercise, Bear Defender, Bear Defender' over our vehicle's PA system. If we didn't see lights coming on in bedrooms then we obviously weren't loud enough, and would start over. The suicide rate amongst West Berliners during these sudden exercises would always spike, as we would find out later, with them believing that the Soviets were invading.

When the wall finally started coming down, we were called out in exactly the same fashion, but this time it was different. We were getting reports of the

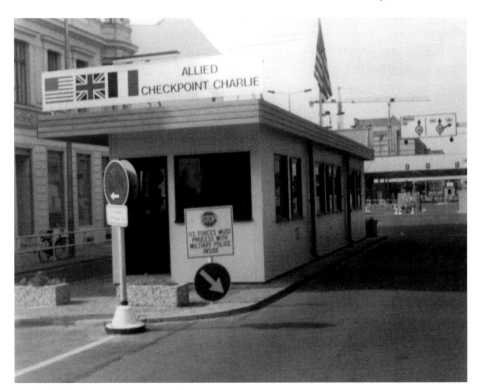

Checkpoint Charlie, where I spent many long days and nights on guard – all of which contributed to my joy when the wall came down!

wall being dismantled and Brigade HQ didn't have a clue what was going on, so RMP were deployed to strategic points to observe and report back. Why RMP? Simply because we were known to go everywhere. Sitting and watching East German border guard activity wasn't uncommon for us... but a tank rolling towards the East German border might just be misinterpreted. It was a truly surreal experience, and I still remember watching East and West Berliners being reunited, friends and families flocking to the walls and crossing points. It was something I'll never forget – the joy, the amazement, the looks on people's faces of pure happiness and relief. I truly felt for them and consider myself incredibly privileged to have witnessed it all at first hand.

In my unit there were lots of guys who had everything that my girlfriend seemed to lack and I worked hard to make sure that I didn't give myself away when we were socialising away from our duties. One night in the corporals' mess, after a particularly hard week, we had colleagues over from Helmstedt, at the other end of the Berlin corridor, to support us with a special event. Our partial social isolation from Army colleagues in our own base made it a pleasing change to get NCOs from another RMP unit to come and join us. With a packed-out barracks, we drank the night away and I spent much of my evening talking to an RMP called Matt. We were of a similar age and background, with the same sense of humour, and it was good to meet somebody from beyond my fishbowl. Plus, he was my type of guy in that he was slightly taller than me, with fair hair and clear blue eyes, and made me laugh more than I did usually. As the evening wore on and the bar started to empty, we found ourselves sat on bar stools at the end, with just a few other guys on the other side. My head was spinning a little and the alarm bells were starting to ring, telling me I had definitely had more than enough booze. I knew it was time to get my head down for the night and make my way back to my room at the other end of the building.

'Right, I'm going to go crash and watch a movie to fall asleep to.' As I stood up to leave, so did Matt, and I heard him grumble about the makeshift room that we had previously set up for around twenty colleagues. I remember laughing at him because they were all sleeping on very uncomfortable camp beds we used on field exercises. A bit 'fresh' in more ways than one. 'Well come and watch some TV for a while,' I said. 'Yeah, alright then,' he replied. Fuelled by the confidence and familiarity of more than a few pints of beer, the door of my room was locked behind us and we were quickly stripped down to our boxers. Keep in mind that the days of being shy for all of us had long gone. The boxers didn't last too much longer before they were cast onto the floor. I was in heaven. Being with another RMP felt safe and we were behind a very secure locked door. It wasn't uncommon for mates to hang out in each other's rooms and typically fall asleep after beers, so no one batted an eyelid when he left my room the next morning looking incredibly hung-over. As far as anyone else was probably concerned, we had been two of the last to leave the bar and had continued drinking in my room. What beasts ... heroes ... men!

Our day of special duties soon started over again, and an hour later, we were amongst the unit stood on parade, ready to begin another long day. Matt returned to Helmstedt that evening, but not before promising, with a knowing and sly smile, to stay in touch. So began a very enjoyable affair, which lasted quite a few months. We'd go out, have drinks, get drunk again, and do the same thing. At the same time, I was dating a German girl, Heidi, to whom I had got chatting after she had stepped on my foot in her high heels at a bar in the city centre. She didn't speak a word of English and our communication actually started by writing on beer mats. I didn't seek her out intentionally as some type of cover to avoid any questions. As I saw more of her, my feelings grew ever stronger and I actually, in a way, fell in love with her because she was absolutely wonderful. To be perfectly honest, the sex with her was fantastic and I was surprised at how strong my feelings for her became. But at the same time, I had very strong feelings for Matt and became very excited at the prospect of each of his visits, although our work made it difficult to plan when we could get together.

Typically, when something is going great, it seems to end all too quickly, and Matt was posted back to the UK. I continued to date Heidi for quite some time and I suspect she thought I might be bisexual. On more than one occasion, the topic of getting together with another couple came up and one of her friends was dating a guy from the Black Watch. We had all met together a few times and somehow, sure enough, we all ended up together after a great night out. It had all been quietly agreed beforehand and so, as guys, we weren't shocked. However, I think we were actually a little shocked at how, all in the same bed, this soldier and I thought nothing of touching each other as well as the girls. This was another reason for me to think that my future in the Army would be fine, or at least not as difficult as I thought it might have been. I also learned that it's generally better to keep my 'interests' away from the sight of my unit, whichever unit that would be in the future. I knew I would have to lead a double life to some extent.

As the months passed, I realised that I would have to split up with Heidi. My time in Berlin was almost up and my posting orders to a new unit would arrive soon. She was incredibly intelligent, lovely, thoughtful and friendly, and much of the relationship felt right. But I understood that my natural pathway in life lay with guys like Matt and my relationship with Heidi had certainly helped keep the wolves from the door. Heidi needed to find a pathway with someone who could

Fellow RMP and I at the Tiergarten Soviet War Memorial as Ceremonial Guards – in battle, all are honoured.

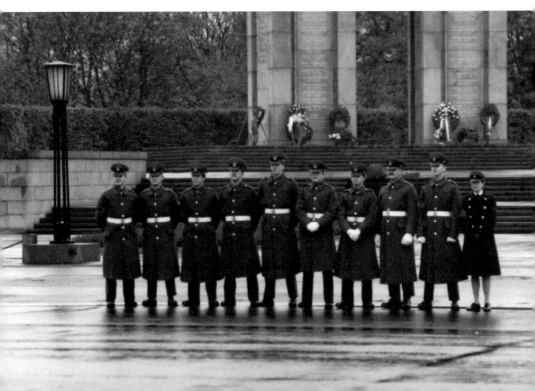

offer much more than I could, and though it was a kindness to let her go, it was the first time I felt such hurt, loss and anguish in my heart. Even to this very day, I often wonder where she is, if is she OK and perhaps married, with kids. I loved her.

Although still in my first posting as Lance Corporal, I was asked if I wanted to be fast-tracked for promotion. I was a bit taken aback at first, but my platoon commander explained that it was felt that I had the potential for more rapid advancement in the RMP. It was a bit uncomfortable for me for a while amongst platoon mates. I had been chosen ahead of others who had been in the Army and RMP longer than I had, but was pleased and excited by the opportunity it offered, so I jumped at the chance.

My 'other' social life took a dive for a while. After Matt and Heidi, I didn't look for new loves or encounters. It was far too risky to go hanging around in any of the gay bars that Berlin was famous for. Just being seen there would end my career – there were no credible excuses. But there was the happy coincidence of my career coming first for a while, so I worked hard and did my best to impress.

Thankfully, we still had adventure training exercises to look forward to. Essentially, they're large team-building trips to remote parts, where you're thrown in with soldiers from various units and trained in rock climbing, abseiling, kayaking, mountain climbing and more. It was definitely not for the faint-hearted and involved two weeks of long days and hard exercise, culminating in a four-day hike with full pack up a mountain range, skirting along its peaks and then down again. I still recall the conditions we were in for that climb: torrential rain, incredible lightning displays at night, and all the time, soaked through to our skin. Everyone was constantly exhausted, but it was fun and we were in it together, regardless of what role we had – an MP looking out for a soldier who was struggling for a few hours, then another soldier looking out for the MP when cramp hit badly. A bond quickly formed between us all. It reinforced our teaching in basic training to look out for one another. This time, the lesson was that it didn't matter what cap badge you had, we were all the same and striving for the same goal. Our only brief periods of respite were at the various lodges we encountered, where a hot meal and thin mattress on the floor were very welcome. In such a cramped space, we were all so close together that I remember waking during the night to discover a fusilier called Mike, who was about 18, tucked in behind me with his arm nestled against my chest. He was fast asleep and I thought nothing of it, and simply drifted off again as quickly as I had woken. Besides, I had noticed him a week earlier and thought for a brief moment that I'd seen a 'knowing look'. The close cuddling felt good.

After finally making our return hike down the mountain, we were all done in. A coach was waiting for us and we scrambled on, eager for the three-hour journey

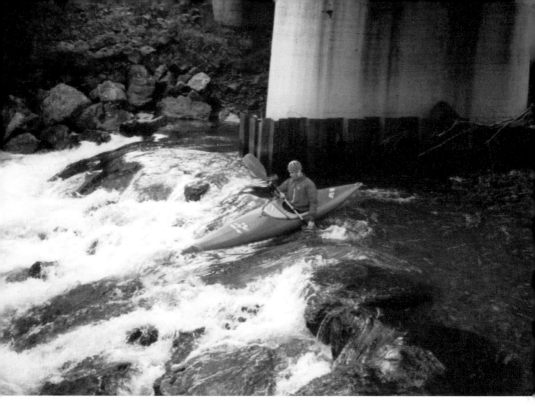

The Army opened the doors for me to try all sorts of sports!

back to our training centre. The same young soldier from the night before found a space next to me at the back. The coach was quiet and most fell asleep quickly. I found a comfy position, half slumped in my seat with kit stowed under my legs. The warmth of the coach was welcoming and I could feel myself drifting off.

I've no idea how long I was asleep for but once again, I woke unexpectedly, this time finding Mike, seemingly asleep, with his head across my stomach. But I now knew different as he had been a couple of seats to my left, and it was definitely a conscious decision to move across and clamber over gear to get to me. Looking around I could see that those nearest to us were still fast asleep and I started thinking of what to do next. I had to give this guy the benefit of the doubt and presume he just wanted to be comfy. I was still a little naive. It became clear he wasn't actually asleep as his arm went around the small of my back and he shuffled to get comfier. I certainly wasn't complaining but at the same time, alarm bells were sounding in my mind. Yet, my hand went to the back of his head and I just started stroking his cropped hair. I knew nothing more could possibly happen as the risk was just way too high. We both seemed content with the situation, though, which he indicated by getting a lot more 'snuggled in' and his fingers gently roaming my lower back under my combat shirt. Neither of us actually slept for the rest of the journey, and although an incredibly sensual experience, we both desperately wanted far more. It was truly frustrating and we knew there would be very little chance of getting more intimate once back at the centre. I wasn't willing to take that risk, much as I wanted to. I didn't see Mike again after that trip but he will always be one of those people in my mind that will never be forgotten. Perhaps I should have let it go a little further at the back of that coach, but I've always been the type that if I did something wrong, I'm guaranteed to get caught out, while others might get off scot-free.

Back in West Berlin, it had been explained to me that my chances of promotion to sergeant were vastly improved if I had served in every part of the Army's geographic 'triangle' of postings at that time: Germany, Northern Ireland and mainland UK. If on that journey I could grab other additional experiences, then that would be even better and would go a long way in promotions selection later. I felt that my time in Berlin had served my career very well, but it was time to broaden my horizons and I volunteered to go to Londonderry. The move came with the rank of corporal. My career was moving on and I could not have been happier with that half of my life. I was just missing being happy about 'me'.

It was a difficult time in Northern Ireland and both soldiers and civilians were being bombed and shot almost weekly. I quickly completed my training for that theatre of operations and was involved in the daily cycle of 'green patrols', where we provided community policing and security patrols from partially armoured vehicles. I say partially, because many lives were still lost to armoured plating

Corporal Darren Ford, South Armagh, 1990, keeping my head down at brew time.

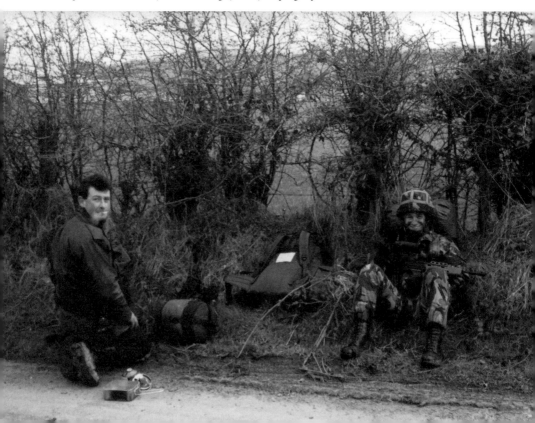

that was simply not up to the job in most cases. Indeed, the Land Rovers we used were often beyond knackered, yet were still somehow trundling along. Even my favourite Land Rover, which I'm standing in front of in the picture in the plate section, is leaning to one side.

There were no trips to the local pub on these tours; your social life was behind the fences, walls and barbed wire. Each of our platoons was in a duty rotation. This meant that we would spend a month on green patrols, a month on border checkpoints and then a month on lighter duties, barracks security and the typical QRF (Quick Reaction Force) tasks. The green patrols I was never a fan of as they were incredibly tedious. After a while, the danger we were in as we roamed notoriously hostile housing estates didn't bother me. You just didn't think about the crap you might end up in. Worrying about what 'could' happen would make you a nervous wreck, and you're no use to anyone in that state. You're a liability.

I preferred going out into the border areas and to the heavily bunkered and armoured checkpoints. The reinforced structures were more for aesthetic and morale purposes really. As I later saw, they were easily destroyed by driving a truck filled to capacity with home-made explosives. We RMP would stand in the road at these checkpoints and stop vehicles, search them if they looked unusually weighted and chat with the occupants. All the while, the checkpoint was manned by an infantry platoon, including supporting cooks. Of course, that wasn't all that we did. We also had intelligence to follow up on and report back any new information that we might have gleaned. We had to look for patterns developing or unusual breaks in patterns. You got to know the locals quickly after speaking to them twice a day, asking about their lives, their jobs, football or whatever it took to get them chatting and having a laugh. I completed two checkpoint tours while at Londonderry.

The first checkpoint I was at was in Belleek, with another RMP colleague from my platoon. Our drive there took around two hours as we took a circuitous route that had already been predetermined. With a quick handover at the checkpoint, the guys from the other platoon were on their way back to barracks. Remembering that usually RMP are always segregated, the squaddies guarding the checkpoint were never easy to chat with, and typically hated MPs. I remember being given very sound advice from a staff sergeant while in Berlin, to always get friendly with the chefs, clerks and medics. An MP might want to be well fed and not have their food spat in, be paid, and then bandaged up when needed. So, with this in mind, I got the chefs laughing, and basically guaranteed we had decent meals! While at the checkpoint I did notice that one of the chefs wasn't very chatty with the squaddies and generally kept to himself. After a few days we noticed that we were getting hot drinks brought out almost every hour, at one point. My colleague complained that he couldn't stop running for a pee every thirty minutes. 'Stop drinking the fucking tea then!' We were even asked what we specifically wanted for dinner after our twelve-hour shift was finished, even though everyone usually made something themselves. It wasn't until later that the checkpoint commander, a sergeant, commented, 'He fancies you …' Initially I wasn't sure how to respond and then quickly asked why he thought that. He explained that before we had arrived days earlier, the squaddies had been taunting the guy and claiming he was gay. This got my back up straight away. I've always hated bullies with a passion and was quick to point out that if I witnessed bullying under his command, then I'd be more than happy to investigate and make arrests. That didn't go down well with the Commander but, let's face it; I wasn't there to be friends with bullies.

Nothing was immediately obvious about the chef in question but, of course, I watched over the coming days, and if you paid close enough attention, there were little details that could easily be missed. His biggest giveaway was his eyes and where they were looking, and that he turned beetroot red if you caught him looking at someone he liked. He certainly wasn't an overtly gay guy, but he ran the risk of being under the spotlight. Should I talk with him about it? Should I ignore and forget?

Two nights later, around 1.00 am, our chef friend was on guard duty at the back of our checkpoint in one of the armoured 'sangars' overlooking the ground to our rear. The shift roster for the squaddies was in easy view and it wasn't difficult to know where he would be, so I headed straight to him. Even in the red light I could see his face turn bright red soon after I walked in. I started talking about why he joined the Army, how long he was going to stay in for and so on. Then I asked if he was gay because I knew someone in RMP who was, and he reminded me of him in some of his mannerisms. There was a long pause and I was about to change the topic when he admitted he was. Now, really speaking, at this point it was my 'duty' to arrest him. Sure, it would have been a great smokescreen for me to have arrested a guy for being gay after admitting it to me, and I could easily have obtained witness statements from the squaddies. The poor guy was almost in tears and my heart went out to him. I daren't risk telling him I was gay, too. I didn't want that coming back to bite me in the backside years later. So, we talked for almost an hour as I explained his giveaway signs and kept reassuring him that he wasn't in trouble (and that our conversation never happened). He seemed happier the next morning and I sensed a change in him. He actually seemed more confident. I still to this day hope the advice I gave him worked out alright.

A few months into my time in Londonderry, I met a friend from my Berlin days, and he recommended I volunteer for the more interesting work of being a Weapons Intelligence Section (WIS) specialist. It was a small unit, mostly of RMP, but included Intelligence and Bomb Disposal personnel. It was much more interesting work and the opportunity to make a real difference to the situation on the ground. I worked in plain clothes, with my partner being a guy from the Intelligence Corps. The section was commanded by a captain from the Royal

Army Ordnance Corps, investigating bombings, shootings and ordnance finds. I had a real sense that I was no longer an ordinary soldier; I was respected, forging a career and doing important work. I spent more and more time in Brigade Headquarters, briefing officers and teams on our findings, and it was on one of these visits that I stumbled across Matt from Berlin. He had been promoted to Corporal and was working in Close Protection, providing a bodyguard service to General Staff. It was dangerous work. We had no time to rekindle our relationship, both being focused very firmly on our work, but it was great to see him again. If nothing else, we tacitly shared the knowledge that people like us can do good, gay or not.

Normally, wherever there were RMP, we had our own bar, but none of us ever liked going there because it was the same old RMP faces, talking about the same old RMP stuff. So we'd all go to the NAAFI, the regular soldiers' bar. One night while at the bar, I caught up with one of the brigade clerks. He was a Geordie and just a year or so older than me. We had a fair few beers, but it was a quiet night and I said I'd turn in early and watch a movie. He asked if he could watch it too, and I agreed! I'm not quite sure how we overcame the natural propensity to dance around the subject, but one way or another, we ended up in bed. Over the months that followed, it happened again a handful of times, but it was high risk. We were

Attending a bombing incident, Armagh, 1992.

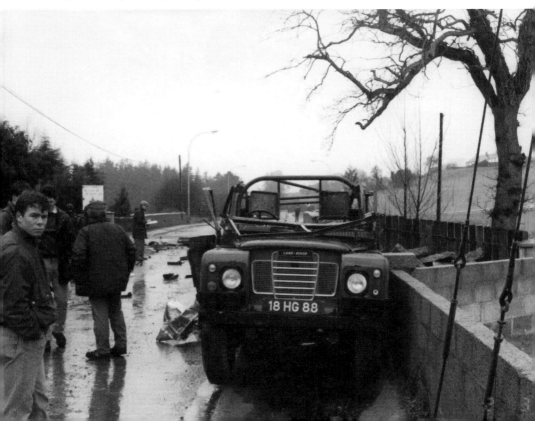

in an operational unit at a very high state of readiness. There were always spare keys for our rooms that a colleague could have got hold of if they wanted to, and the barracks we were accommodated in had paper-thin walls and creaky iron beds. It was risky, but my life had become very work-focused and I needed something to add a bit of joy here and there. In part to keep a smokescreen, I started dating a new RMP corporal who was living in female quarters in our barracks. When I asked if she was on the green patrols, her answer stopped me dead in my tracks: 'the Special Investigation Branch'. Most people might think I should have found some excuse to not get anywhere near her, but the truth is, she was fun and surely, no one would even think I was gay! It didn't last long, though, and we parted on good terms.

In January 1993, I left Northern Ireland and returned to Germany. It was Dusseldorf this time, and regular patrolling. Compared to my work in Northern Ireland, it was incredibly dull and lacked the purpose and importance of my weapons intelligence work. I was only there for eight months, but it dragged, and my spare time was particularly dull, until I discovered a video store that had gay porn. One of the great things about being an RMP was that you were the least likely person to be stopped and questioned, and highly unlikely to be searched by the squaddies when coming back onto base, and for a while I enjoyed watching the likes of Helmut and Hanz, who always seemed to be 'here to mend your washing machine'!

I rarely went into the RMP bar in Dusseldorf but one night I thought I'd give it a go. I'd had eight consecutive night patrols and I'm rubbish at sleeping during daylight hours, so was pretty exhausted. One beer led to another and I was more than tipsy. RMPs are good at looking after one another after drinking. The consequences of poor behaviour after alcohol were serious and we needed to watch each other's backs. Sam was one of our first tour NCOs. He had a bit of a boy-next-door look about him and as I bade goodnight to the fellow drunks, he volunteered to 'put me down', as he was leaving anyway. So I hobbled off my bar stool and was supported back to my room in the barracks. Dressed in my off-shift combats and boots, he got me out of my jacket and olive drab shirt, and wrestled off my boots, all the while chatting away to me and saying 'You've been working hard, Corporal, and needed to blow off a bit of steam.' At this point I thought he would stop, but he didn't, and instead pushed me back onto my bed. By this time, I was in my boxer shorts, laid on my bed with my back to the door in the semi-dark, with a huge boner trying desperately to escape from my boxers. I heard the door close and was surprised to hear it locked from the inside. I turned around, a little confused and expecting Sam to have gone. He hadn't. He then came to sit next to me and said nothing for what seemed like an eternity. Without a word, he quickly undressed, took down my boxers and got in next to me. It's amazing how quickly you can sober up!

To this day I wonder about those senior officers who had the arrogance to believe that gay men and women were a half handful of people in the Armed Forces, in roles that didn't matter. Even though it was illegal to be gay, we were everywhere, quietly getting on with doing our bit the best we could. The lesbians were more obvious than the very discreet and closeted gays, by far. I got the impression that there was a queen bee in every barracks; the stereotype would have been a big butch girl, but the reality I know was very different. There were all sorts of us, all people I'm proud of, not just for their service, but for the complex lives they lived … with the constant worry that their career could be over if their sexuality were discovered. How did we manage with that kind of stress on top of everything else?

Towards the end of my time in Dusseldorf I became friendly with another RMP called Pete. He was a gym bunny and spent way too much time on his fitness, but every so often he'd go into Dusseldorf centre to blow out the cobwebs. He seemed to know good places to go, which was generally away from the routes we took each day patrolling for squaddies. One Saturday, as we left a bar, we took a right turn into the 'red light district'. It was a little after midnight and after sharing a few racy stories about nights out on the town, he announced: 'I'm really horny and I need sex.'

The best I could say was, 'Oh, right mate, you go for it,' and I started thinking where the nearest taxi would be. He started chatting up a prostitute he had picked out and asked, 'How much for both of us?'

I was taken aback, but before I could back out, he had paid for us both. Clearly, Pete was interested in more than the girl because it was in every way a threesome. As far as I knew, if you paid for a prostitute then that was what you were there for … not looking at me, touching, and then kissing. I certainly wasn't complaining, though! From the moment we walked out, it was back to the 'straight lads' kind of chat. We never spoke about what Pete and I did together; it was forgotten about and became one of those stories that reinforced our straight credentials. Being in the room next to mine at our barracks, there were many times I thought something might have happened while we were sat watching TV together. But it never did.

Within six months, our Dusseldorf barracks was closed, as part of cost saving, I guess, and all of the occupying units were moved to Rheindahlen, a very large garrison town with, I'm sure, lots of opportunity if I wanted to find it … but also, lots of gossip and high risk. I hated it there.

Not long after arriving there, though, I returned to the UK on compassionate grounds. My parents' marriage had hit the rocks, the family situation was pretty desperate and my little brother was struggling to cope. Although prepared to wreck the careers and lives of gay men and women, the British Armed Forces were very good at compassionately looking after families in crisis, as long as they were straight.

So my first time back in mainland UK, and to begin with, it felt like a very strange existence. I'd been away for many years and the normality of my home life was in stark contrast to my time in Germany and Northern Ireland. I reconnected with friends and started getting a bit more adventurous in my social life. And so

I began to live a double life. During most of my working week I had my military life, an exemplary and well-respected RMP NCO, on a career fast track, and on my days off, close to the family home, searching for friendships and lovers.

I've generally always found it easy to make new friends, although I admit that nowadays, I can detect signs of a moron from afar and tend not to place much trust in people. But generally, RMP and civvy police have always got on well together. It was while on our usual patrols out of Telford that I met Rob, a civvy copper who had a slightly Mediterranean look about him and who made me laugh. He was seeing a girl locally and we became friends. I'd sometimes go over to his house to watch a movie, or for him to show off his homebrew factory in his spare bedroom and sample some of the oddly tasting stuff he was making. He'd often ask me over for drinks when his fiancé was away and always suggest I could stay in the spare room if I got too drunk. He explained I was good company and it wasn't like he could go crawling around Telford bars, being a copper and all. I did go for beers quite a few times but never stayed over; a taxi back to barracks was cheap, and anyway, why bother staying? It wasn't like anything was going to happen with him. He was just a good mate looking out for me.

I ended up dating a civilian guy from the Wirral, where I'm from. It was an amazing experience, with an eerie sense of normality after meeting him in a nightclub in Chester, of all places. James was my first proper boyfriend and I finally felt I was beginning to understand what my Army lifestyle was denying me. It wasn't a relationship that lasted beyond six months, but for the most part, I enjoyed our time together. He just had some serious issues that I wasn't able to cope with. Through James, I met a friend of his called Liam, and after a little time, we became close and saw each other at every opportunity. He lived with his parents and didn't seem to have much going on in his life, but I was searching for a relationship and he was in the right or wrong place at the time. It was what I'd call a honeymoon relationship, because we only saw each other twice a week. It's a lesson I carry with me, that there are things you don't see when you're not with somebody the whole time.

Fairly early on in our relationship, my regimental sergeant major (RSM) told me that I had been selected to go for a six-month exchange tour in Australia. Not too bad really, being picked from around 2,800 MPs worldwide!

'Can I think about it, sir?'

'What do you mean, think about it, you wanker? … I'll give you two days.'

I wanted to speak to Liam about it, which he reluctantly agreed to but on the condition that we took a holiday to The Gambia first – which I was to pay for. It seemed a strange destination for us, and certainly not a gay metropolis, so I knew I'd be able to relax and we could be a 'normal' couple. As we were about to land at Banjul Airport, the pilot announced that there had been a peaceful military coup and the country was continuing as normal. I was probably more relaxed about that than most of the tourists on the plane. A couple of days after we arrived, I met

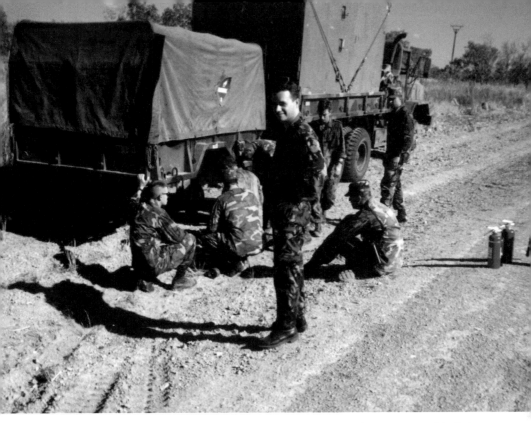

Above and below: Corporal Darren Ford, Exercise Longlook, Australia, 1995 – an escape and 'quiet' before the storm.

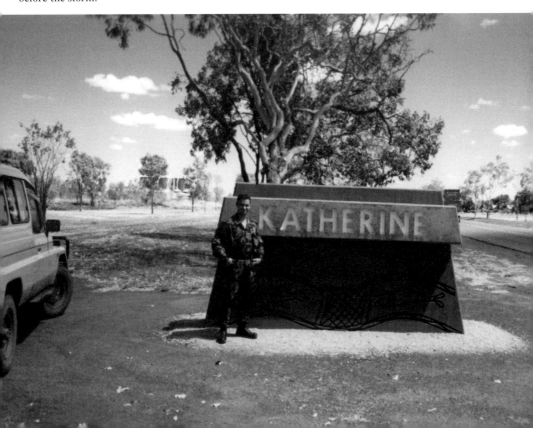

the 'unsinkable' Craig Jones at the beach bar at the Senegambia Hotel. It is an ordinary truth that servicemen can always spot each other in a way that is much more accurate than a gaydar. It was very apparent to me that we were both cut from the same cloth, and it was also obvious that we were both on holiday with our boyfriends. There was a comedy moment at the bar of 'you show me yours and I'll show you mine', and glances at ID cards were exchanged. Mine was, of course, a warrant card, which widened his grin; we were, quite literally, partners in crime. When the ban was lifted years later, this irrepressible officer fought the corner of serving gay men and women like a tiger. I can only imagine that there must be admirals, generals and air marshals still picking buckshot out of their backsides!

Sadly, the holiday was over all too quickly and I found myself in Australia. The whole six months went by in an uneventful way from a gay point of view, although I did venture out to some of the gay bars in Sydney, so long as they were off the beaten track, as such.

After my Australian jaunt, my unit was put on notice to transition to the NATO operation in Bosnia. I was the senior radio operator and would go in the first wave to Gornji Vakuf, and I deployed on 23 December 1995. We arrived with

Relaxing on the beach in Australia.

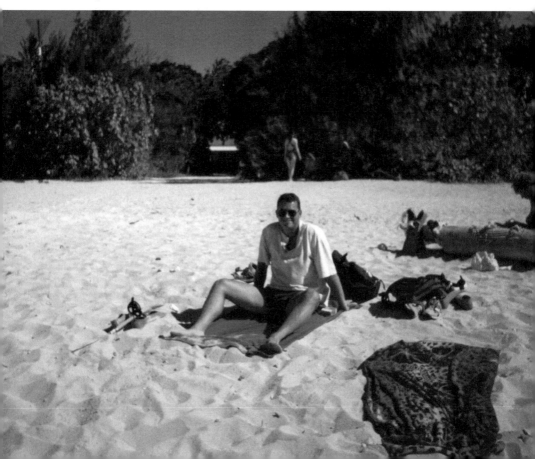

blue United Nations berets, but switched overnight to a NATO operation and replaced them with our distinctive scarlet red berets. The first two months were unremarkable as we established our presence.

Suddenly, out of the blue, I was called in to speak to my RSM, who explained I had to return to the UK to face investigation. He said material had been found in my barrack room back home, where they were taking the opportunity to do some renovations while the unit was overseas. 'Oh shit,' I thought. I did have a couple of gay magazines and a letter from Liam under my mattress, and although we never used names when writing to each other, there were still risks. It wasn't a deliberate search; it was just purely bad luck. The humiliating part was having my personal items searched, having to quickly pack a bag and then get escorted in a Land Rover accompanied by two RMP SIB NCOs. I managed to get a call to Liam and we agreed a story that he was a lifelong family friend and not 'out' to his parents – I'd been keeping the items for him.

To my shock, within an hour of getting back to our base, the two SIB officers went straight to Liam's house, where his mum and dad were, and interviewed him. Within another hour, they had their witness statement. In all honesty, I don't think that these officers actually cared whether I was gay, straight, bisexual, lesbian, alien or whatever. It was a break from the front line; they had their statement and were on their way home, having resolved a seemingly uncomplicated case. I suspected that I knew them, and they knew I had dated two women from SIB.

While this was going on, I got regular visits from my mate Rob, who came to see how I was. Gossip travels fast in police circles, and he was genuinely concerned and offered to catch up with beers. I explained that my head wasn't with it right now. After he had gone, my RSM told me I couldn't have police social visits as it wasn't 'appropriate'. Well, that was bullshit. I told Rob, of course, and he just laughed.

I realised that the longer I stayed away from my unit in Bosnia, the worse the impact would be, and within a week I was returning to Gornji Vakuf.

In my Army career there have been a few moments of which I am proud. My return to my unit in Bosnia is one of those. To the men and women in my unit, I had been tainted by being accused of being queer and subjected to substantial challenges, but I walked back into camp with my head held so high I was touching the clouds. I could see my mates grinning ear to ear at my lack of shame or sense of guilt.

I will always remember a close friend's comment in the mess that night: 'I don't really give a fuck whether you are gay or not, but I just loved the way you walked in front of everyone as though saying "Fuck you, you bunch of twats".' Happy days.

Our tour in Bosnia was short and I returned to Telford with my unit, where my CO reminded me that I was on the fast track for promotion and that there was

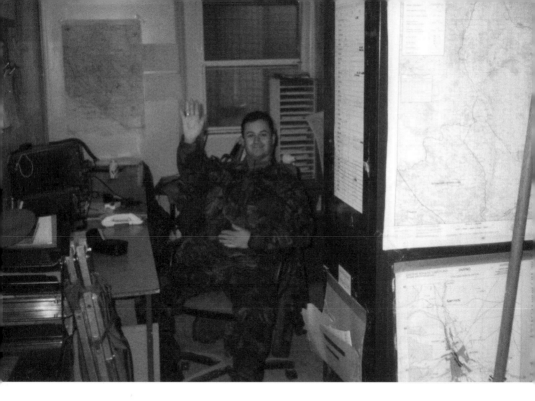

Above: In the office at our IFOR base in Tomislavgrad, Bosnia, 1996.

Below: I stumbled across Malaysian soldiers as part of IFOR and exchanged photos not far from Tomislavgrad, Bosnia.

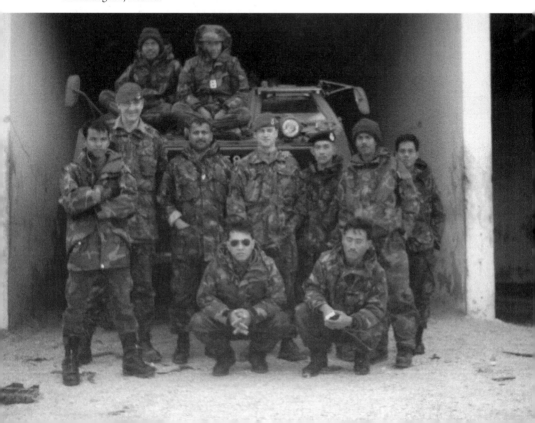

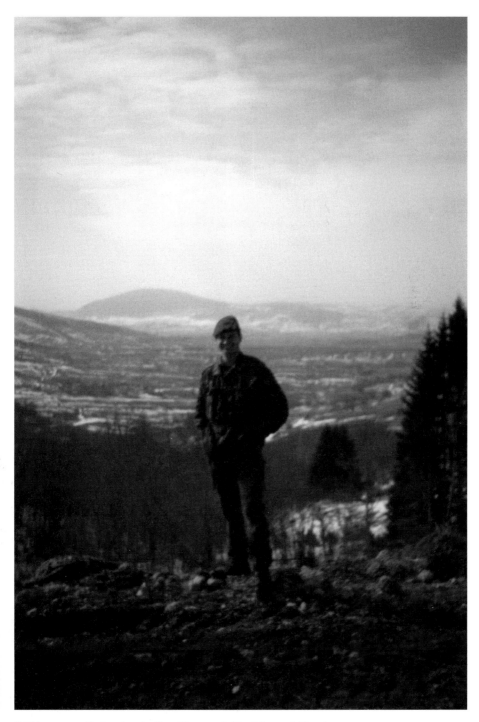

Still have to smile, laugh at it all and be proud. Tomislavgrad, Bosnia.

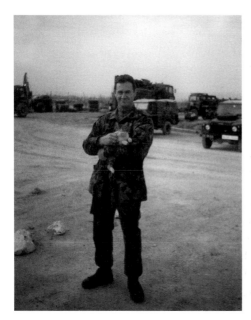 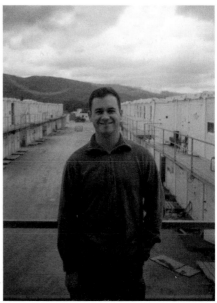

Above left and right: Pictured with our unit cat, just before I left Bosnia in 1996 and in our temporary accommodation. Had I got away with it?

an opportunity with a Territorial Army unit, 160 (Wales) Brigade Provost Unit in Cardiff, and with it, I would be promoted to sergeant. It seemed like a comedy: one minute I'm being chucked out, next minute I'm being promoted.

Leaving my unit was a wrench. In the most discrete way, some of my closest friends were beginning to know that I was gay, but they didn't care. The military was changing, but, forgive the pun, from the bottom up. Ordinary soldiers did not share the discomfort of senior officers and most had little issue with having gay men in their midst, as long as they were good soldiers. Rob was happy I'd gained the promotion, but sad too that I was moving down to Cardiff. He was a good guy and little did I know that I wouldn't see him again until after I'd left the Army.

As soon as I arrived in Cardiff I discovered that my unit had not completed its obligatory two weeks' deployment, which would result in them losing a lot of pay, and the unit was already at risk of closure. As the permanent staff instructor, it fell on me to pull this unit out of its shitty decline, so I set to the task. I started calling other RMP TA units to see if I could get help around my unit's two-week deployment. After calling several with no luck, I tried a unit in Northern Ireland. Matt, whom I knew from Berlin, answered the phone! They were going to Gibraltar and had space. I remember it as a very enjoyable trip. In my unit I became a legend, having pulled a rabbit out of the hat. All I can say is that it was a win-win situation. There was no chance of Matt and me resuming our previous exploits. We were just too high profile in our units and the focus was constantly on us, with never a moment's peace.

Back home in the Wirral, things were going badly from all angles. After almost two years, Liam still had no job and our lives were diverging fast. He was making no effort in life and was still living with his parents. He started becoming quite resentful of the fact that I'd been promoted, that I'd been to Australia and had recently got a 'new' second-hand car. He seemed bitter that he had to give a witness statement to get me out of trouble and he kept mentioning it with an air of menace. I tried to break with him and he quickly resorted to extortion, his immediate response being, 'If you don't see me, I'm telling the Army.' That started in August 1996, soon after my arrival in Cardiff, and continued until 25 December. The aim of his blackmail was to force me to see him whenever I had free time. It had become an abusive relationship and I hated him for it. In an act of defiance that brought matters to a conclusion, I spent Christmas Day with family, and then on the morning of the 26th, I had a phone call around 7.00 am: it was Liam, raging threats down the line. He finished the call by saying, 'I've decided I'm telling the Army, fuck you.'

I pleaded with him: 'Look, don't do this. This is going to ruin my career.'

'Well, you should have thought about that yesterday when you ignored me.'

He put the phone down, and I rang him back straight away. I had reached the end of my tolerance and something snapped. 'You know what? Do what the fuck you like. I don't give a fuck anymore,' and I put the phone down.

I knew he would be straight on the phone to RMP Telford, my old unit, which I'd left only a few months earlier. I started shaking, sitting in the living room of my rented flat in the Wirral. I started crying, stopped long enough to make a brew and then burst into tears again. My head was swimming with what was about to happen, what had gone on, what my future would be and how I could possibly face anyone ever again. I knew he'd make that call and be enjoying his moment. Twenty minutes later, he rang me back, and said, 'There you go, I've called them. They're going to be calling you soon.' He hung up and that was the last time I spoke to him.

My mind is still hazy about what happened next but I do remember wishing I wasn't there anymore. I didn't have the energy physically or mentally to keep on going. I wanted to sleep and never wake up again. I was done.

I started running a bath and then my mum rang. To this day, I've no idea why she just happened to call my phone at such an early time. Intuition? I don't remember the conversation at all, but it was brief. I do remember getting the sharpest knife from the kitchen and taking it to the bathroom with me, and then sitting on the edge of the bath waiting for it to fill. It seemed to be taking forever. I remember thinking that the water had to be quite hot for what I was about to do. That's what I'd learned while being in the RMP, from attending suicides. Finally, the bath was full and the water so hot I could barely dip my hand in it. This would do.

As I started to strip, I was startled by a hammering at my front door. I paused to see if they would go away but no, whoever it was was persistent and didn't seem to be taking silence as an answer to bugger off. Outside, I found my mum, stepmum, dad and two of my sisters anxiously waiting. How much time had passed? Why were they here? What had I said on the phone? I had lost everything and their swift reaction on that day saved me. I just burst into tears once they all got into the living room. I can still see my dad scurrying around the flat searching for something … returning a few minutes later with the knife in his hand and discretely putting it back in the kitchen drawer. My dad could be a tough man. He didn't look angry; he looked scared. I really don't recall what happened over the next few days other than I was staying with dad. It's simply a blank in my memory.

My CO was a very decent bloke; he was an ex-RSM, old school, but a damn good guy. I obviously had to tell him what had gone on as he would soon have found out from my old unit in Telford. In the aftermath, he made an appointment for me to see the medics at Dale Barracks. As I cried down the phone to this very senior and experienced officer, he told me not to worry about anything. All that could be done would be done. Very soon afterwards, I went to Dale Barracks in Chester to see the medical officer, who prescribed Valium. Then she rang my CO. He confirmed what had happened and he and the medical officer agreed on a long period of leave. Most importantly, the medical officer told the SIB that I was unfit to interview – a great kindness.

When the time came for me to face my fate, I met with my old CO, who was also the ultimate MP in our division as Provost Marshal. I recounted the turn of events, leaving nothing out. 'Well, I appreciate you being honest with me. These are the options we've got now: you either deny and you'll be investigated and then go to court martial, or I can put you forward for court martial today because you've admitted in front of the RSM and me that the evidence is there. The other alternative is that you ask to resign and serve twelve months' notice.' It was immediately apparent that I was being given the chance to retain my rank, get my red book and keep my pension. I would need to sign to say that I had requested to leave the Army, but amidst a range of unwelcome options, it seemed the very best of a bad job.

After a couple of weeks, I returned to look after my TA unit in Cardiff and gathered them together to explain what had happened and what was going to happen now. To my surprise, they didn't give a shit that I was gay. Some had already guessed anyway, and weren't fazed by this 'surprise' revelation. Most were angry that I had to leave them eventually. Their little unit had been turned from the brink of closure to one that had a good role to play, and was gaining strength each month.

The camaraderie had improved dramatically and recruitment was up. I still remember them talking together after our meeting about a huge leaving party. Talk about prior planning! As it happens, my leaving party was indeed huge, with friends travelling from other units as well as some associates from the police forces I'd worked with and got to know well. It was a night to remember … almost as much as the hangover next day!

The weird thing is, I would not fucking change a thing. Yes, I had to lead a double life. Yes, I had a breakdown. Yes, there were lots of tears and mental anguish, but I finally exorcised my blackmailer with as much dignity as I could manage. It was a massive relief. I was angry

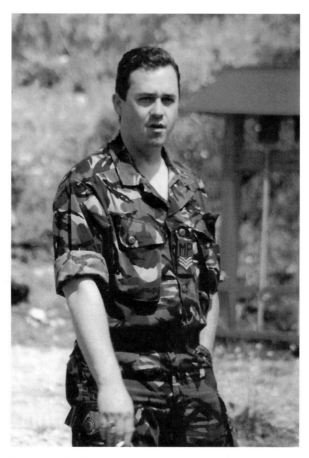

Permanent Staff Instructor at 160 (W) BPU RMP (V) - taking time out briefly at firing ranges in Gibraltar.

at the turn of events, for sure, and to some extent, I still am. Of a twenty-two-year commitment, I managed just over half, but would have been very proud to have had the chance to serve my time and climb that promotion ladder as quickly as had been apparently planned. But I survived, and these dreadful events made me the man I am today – and I'm quite happy with me.

The experience with Liam did have a lasting impact, though, and even after later loves, I still struggle to place a lot of trust in partners or let anyone get too close. I have, eventually, trusted a partner. My last three partners let me down badly in various ways. When I visualise how my heart would look, it has four massive scars slashed into it, and, although recovered and healed, I'm not sure I would open it to another so easily.

I know it's something I should force myself to do, in a way. But my mind keeps reminding me of what can happen when you let people into your world and share little secrets. Oddly enough, my friends today confide in me so much, and I know they find it a little frustrating when I don't give as much in return.

I didn't go back to punish Liam after I left the forces, although I was tempted to find some way at times. Although I would have gained some small amount of satisfaction, it wasn't in my nature to be such a little shit as he was. So I was silent. Two Christmases after leaving, a greetings card addressed to me arrived at my mother's home. It was from Liam, and inside he had a written a long letter of apology, begging for forgiveness and including his mobile number. I never acknowledged it and just threw it in the bin. I didn't want to remember him anymore and didn't care that he felt such guilt. He continued to send a Christmas card, with letter and phone number, for the next six years or so.

I have often imagined what would happen if I saw him in the street here in Manchester, where he knew I had moved to. I'd stop him, ask if he remembered me, make sure he did and then walk away.

Do you recall Rob, the civvy copper? Years later, I was on holiday with friends in Gran Canaria when, in one of the hundred or so gay bars, I got a tap on the shoulder. I turned to see Rob, beaming at me, and I hugged him hard straight away. It turned out that he had kept an eye on me from afar while I was in Cardiff through his counterparts in South Wales Police, who were also in my unit as RMP TA guys. He had followed what I had been going through. He also explained how he had left his fiancé, sold his house, left the police and was now a tour guide in Gran Canaria, living with his boyfriend. Damn! Now I understood why he kept asking me to stay over when we had a beer night!

I've often been asked whether I had any regrets from that period of my life. I don't. The only regret I do have that plays on my mind almost every day, is that I lost touch with so many amazing and supportive people who were solid friends. I only wish I knew where they were now.

I'm not envious of gay soldiers who serve today. In fact, I'm incredibly happy for them. I hope they are as lucky as I was to serve with brilliant people in exciting jobs. Getting to where our Armed Forces are today was quite a journey, and it needed people like me and many others to throw themselves on the fire along the way! I am thankful, though, that the compassion of men and women whose respect I had won enabled me to leave the Army with much of my dignity intact. I know that many others were sadly not as lucky as I was, and they lost far more than I did.

Chapter 7

This Queer Angel
Lieutenant Elaine Chambers
Queen Alexandra's Royal Army Nursing Corps

I first voiced an interest in serving Queen and country back in 1979, but the seed was firmly planted on 25 February 1974, when BBC2 broadcast an extraordinarily brave yet controversial drama. I'll never know why I was allowed to stay up late to watch it, especially as it was preceded, unusually, by a warning of adult content. Aged only 13 and raging with hormonal confusion, I experienced the first profoundly disturbing and erotic introduction to my sapphic leanings. With my mum and nain (pronounced 'nine', the Welsh word for grandmother), I watched a short play in a series called *Second City Firsts*. One of the actors was a very young Alison Steadman, in an early role.

The play, called *Girl*, was written by James Robson and focused on a Women's Royal Army Corps barracks. As the story unfolded I was totally unprepared for the flashback scene showing two women in bed, clearly naked. Although thankfully our front room wasn't very well lit, this being the era of filament light bulbs, I was convinced that my beetroot flushes were not only visible but palpable. I was burning up, scanning Mum's and Nain's faces for any sign that they knew how I was feeling. The intensity of my reaction made me feel certain

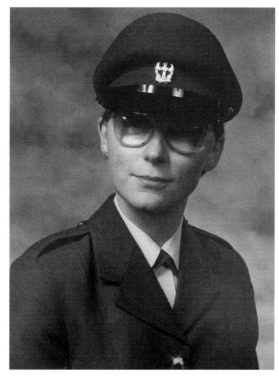

Private Chambers, April 1982.

that they must have known. The flutter of butterflies in my stomach was overwhelming, and as the play continued, it became clear that two of the four characters were unashamedly lesbian. I was aware of the tension in the front room. In fairness to Mum and Nain, they didn't make too much of a fuss and just tutted and sighed when the 'fruitier' moments occurred. Although ultimately quite a sad story, there was some humour and quite near-the-knuckle language, which was beyond my innocent ken. But the scene that literally blew my world wide open came towards the end of the story, involving Myra Frances (playing serially seducing Corporal Chrissie Harvey) and Alison Steadman (the raw recruit Jackie Smithers). After holding one another tightly, Jackie asked Chrissie if she would miss her when she'd gone back to Civvy Street. After Chrissie said yes, they kissed passionately, not once, but twice. This – not Anna Friel's often cited but comparatively tame effort in the Channel 4 soap *Brookside* – was the first lesbian kiss ever to be broadcast on British TV … and I had witnessed it! I didn't realise it at the time, but the setting of a training depot had subliminally crept into my subconscious.

It was almost on a whim that I visited the Central London Recruiting Depot one day in late summer 1980. I was 19 years old and had decided to see if it was possible to enlist in the Women's Royal Army Corps as a driver. A flashback to Myra Frances, so smart and sassy in her uniform, set the dream in motion. I had no better ideas for a career … why not give it a try? The recruiting sergeant ran through my details and sighed. 'Everyone who applies to join the WRAC wants to be a driver and there's a two-year waiting list,' he said. 'You've got A levels, so why don't you join the QAs instead?' Two years? A lifetime! Having never heard of the QAs, I was duly sent away clutching a set of glossy brochures and printed lists of current pay rates to peruse. It turned out that the QAs stood for Queen Alexandra's Royal Army Nursing Corps; apparently, I was destined to become a nurse, not a driver.

I joined in 1982 and had the great fortune to be trained in what was called a modular style, with small classes and brilliant support. This was the era shortly before a much lauded new method, Project 2000, was being launched throughout the NHS nationwide. We went to Woolwich to do our six-week introductory nursing course, which would set us up for what was to come over the next three years. It was during this period that we were finally told where we'd be posted. At the age of 21, three years seemed like an eternity, and seeing it all written down for the first time was quite daunting. I got a posting to Rinteln in Germany for the first eighteen months and then back to the Cambridge Military Hospital, Aldershot for the second eighteen months.

The thought of making it through three years of training to become a QA was just phenomenal. The corps can trace its heritage back to Florence Nightingale, who was instrumental in lobbying for the support of female military nurses. As a

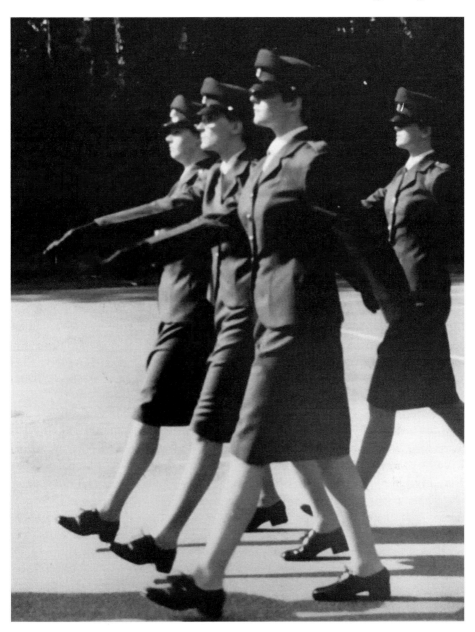

Passing out parade, QATC Aldershot, April 1982.

student nurse I was neither brilliant nor awful – I loved the practical side of things and really enjoyed learning new skills, such as different dressing techniques, how to give injections, take blood samples, pass nasogastric tubes, insert catheters and the like, but it wasn't until we did our three weeks in maternity that I began to be genuinely excited at the possibility that I had found the specialism for me. Had I stayed in the Army, midwifery would have been my chosen post-graduate course of study, but sadly, it was not to be.

Sadie and I had joined up at the same time. She had lovely pale blue eyes, was rather foxy and naughty, and her voice was quite deep. I liked her sense of humour and found myself trying to amuse and generally impress her. After we'd completed our six weeks' basic training we were all posted to the Queen Elizabeth Military Hospital at Woolwich. We were billeted in four-bedded rooms and I was sharing with Sadie, Ally and Tiff. As the weeks passed I found myself feeling more and more attracted to Sadie. One day, we were sitting facing one another across a fairly small table, ostensibly revising for our end of course assessments. By this time she had started seeing a massive guy who was a physiotherapist, very much a muscle-bound hunk. We were knocking back cans of Woodpecker cider and had cassettes playing in the background, and found ourselves talking about first kisses. We were looking very closely at one another. Yet somehow, I genuinely do not know *how*, I knew she'd been involved with a woman during our basic training! After what felt like hours of flirting and skirting around same-sex attraction, we finally kissed. In that instant, my life changed irrevocably. After that we only had a couple of chances to spend time alone together before I was posted to Germany in June 1982, and that was when we went to stay at Sadie's mum's house. By then I was becoming inwardly obsessive about her and I was indeed whatever the name was that could be used to describe a woman who loved women.

I was dreading going to Rinteln, leaving Sadie to be posted elsewhere in the UK. We'd had a really enjoyable few weeks together and our relationship had developed. Sadie was far more sanguine about it all. We wrote to one another a few times after we'd been posted but deep down, I knew it would probably never amount to anything more. Out in Germany, squaddies were always on the lookout for women to come to their dances and their mess balls. When an invitation went up on the billet notice boards, competition would be fierce, particularly if there was a restricted number of invites available.

On one occasion there was an opportunity to be picked up and taken by coach to Sennelager, a town with a military base about an hour's drive away, for a Royal Scots Dragoon Guards ball. I put my name down at the top of the list, and it was closely followed by those of all my friends. This was one do we weren't going to miss! When we arrived we were 'piped in' to the huge hall by a very handsome young soldier in full kilted regalia – all very exciting. I was seated between two officers. The chap to my right had a very Scottish sounding name but spoke with the plummiest of BBC accents, which was a little disconcerting. Angus was an unmitigated prat: totally pretentious, arrogant and generally up himself. By the end of the delicious meal and the excellent demonstration of Highland dancing, Angus seemed quite smitten with me. He was about to ask me onto the dance floor when a skinny young lad with dark brown hair and pale blue eyes suddenly stepped between us. 'Er, would yer like ter have a wee dance? – Aw, gaw on, yer know yer want tae!' His lilting Scottish accent, cheeky grin and the fact that he seemed a teensy bit pissed made him so much more appealing and real than that stuffed shirt prig. I took the lad's hand and walked to the dance floor, saying, 'I'd love to, thanks.'

Joe was celebrating his twenty-first birthday and was fairly well oiled by the time we met. We didn't even kiss, but we exchanged phone numbers. I wasn't really expecting to hear from him again but I did, and we began dating. Luckily for us, my good friend Amy had started seeing a friend of Joe's and this began a series of double dates. Joe was from Stirling and I understood his accent fairly well but he had a disconcerting habit of using Cockney rhyming slang. He would say things that left me completely baffled, such as, 'Och, me clathes are killing me.' I'd have to work out what he was saying and then translate it from the Cockney: 'Oh Elaine, my clothes pegs are killing me!' – clothes pegs = legs … 'Oh, are your legs aching, Joe?' 'Aye, hen. I've been playing footie all weekend!'

Despite my straight credentials being in good shape due to having Joe with me, at the usual round of NAAFI discos and other soirées, rumours began. One particular episode left me seething with rage. Another student, Wendy, was sitting up talking with me one night and the conversation came around to same-sex attraction. I was initially very wary as I hadn't for a moment seen it coming. I gradually felt as if I could trust her and having told her a bit about my own experience, I felt oddly relieved. Only a few days later, I was out drinking in a German-owned pub right outside the main entrance to the hospital with my best friends. One of them told me that Wendy had been telling anyone who would listen that they should be careful never to find themselves alone in a lift with me! I couldn't believe how stupid and trusting I'd been – would I never learn? I went to the loo and smashed my clenched fist through the small opaque window. Luckily, the noise of the other drinkers and the music from the jukebox had covered the sound of my destructive outburst. As I'd already confided in my friends about my confusion, they felt I should just ignore it and concentrate on making it all work with Joe.

After Rinteln came the second eighteen months of training. This saw a return to Aldershot, where I'd done my basic training. The Cambridge Military Hospital, known as CMH, was where I would spend the next two and a half years. This wonderful place served as the area's main general hospital and 70 per cent of patients were civilians with no military connections. We were immensely proud to hear rumours that ambulance crews were often begged to come to us rather than the nearest NHS hospital. With the benefit of hindsight, I can honestly say that this was one of the happiest times of my life. The incredible people I was working with, the friendships that I forged and the wonderful social life all led to the most

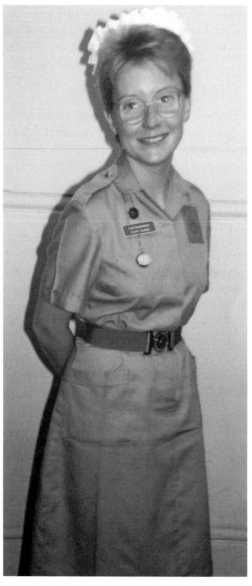

Newly qualified Staff Nurse Chambers, autumn 1985.

incredible feeling of belonging and personal satisfaction at having decided to follow this profession. I had a real sense of purpose and the possibility of a long, stable and promising career ahead of me. Towards the end of my time there I was successful in my application to become a commissioned officer.

Having already completed my basic training as a private, officer training was a doddle. Apart from one other Army nurse from 'the ranks', a lovely sergeant called Jen Ritchie, whom I knew through having briefly worked with her before, all the others in our officer intake were direct entry from the NHS. We would find ourselves being consulted about how best to bull shoes, get the dreadful white number two blouses ironed correctly (they had the most awful pleats front and back, which were total bastards to iron to a satisfactory standard to pass inspection), and shape our grey berets into something that didn't look too much like a flying saucer or a large felt pancake. We'd often smile at the indignant reactions of the others to being chastised ever so politely if items of uniform weren't quite meeting the required standard. 'Was the iron switched on, ladies?' One thing that I did enjoy just as much was my second passing out parade in early December 1986. It is impossible for me to convey the sense of pride and belonging, knowing that your family are straining to pick you out as your platoon rounds the corner onto the drill square on such a momentous day.

My first posting as Sister Chambers was to be to Catterick, North Yorkshire. I was frankly gutted, having hoped, after nearly three years back in the UK,

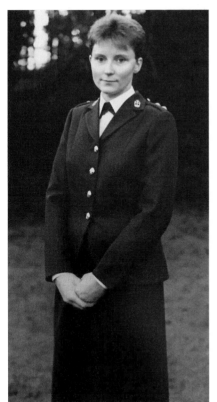 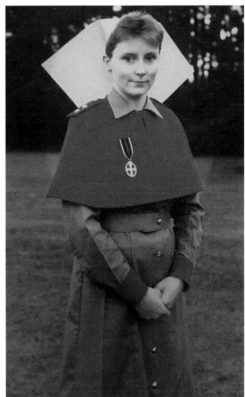

Above left: Newly commissioned Lieutenant Chambers, 1986.

Above right: Sister Chambers, 1986.

it might be time for a more desirable overseas deployment. Jen had got Hannover, and was equally disappointed as her boyfriend was based in the north of England. We dared wonder if we should push our luck and ask whether we might swap. We were the only two Army trained nurses, so had a similar background. Amazingly, our request was granted. Hindsight being 20/20, I have often wondered how things might have turned out had I just accepted my originally intended posting to Catterick, but if I hadn't have asked to swap, I wouldn't have got to know one of my best friends, Gail, and my life would have been so much poorer without her.

When we first went to Germany, many of us hadn't lived far away from our family homes and when crises occurred we had to support each other emotionally. Being away in Germany, before easy instant communication through emails, social media, iPads and mobiles, meant we became really close as we couldn't easily ring home. We had little choice but to rely upon one another for succour, support and advice whenever problems arose. Such close interdependence creates deep bonds that last forever. This was at a time when the Cold War threat was very real too, so there was a sense that life might be fragile. Knowing that the sheer weight and numbers of East German and Russian forces, who were very close by, could easily destroy our tactically superior weaponry within a very short period of time probably contributed to our 'eat, drink and be merry, for tomorrow we may die' attitude. There were a few pretty serious discussions about what the reality of an invasion would be. The knowledge that we were on the wrong side of the very wide river Weser was quite alarming. And we knew we would be expected to stay with any patients unable to be evacuated. Plus the Army Air Corps based at Detmold, a mere eight minutes' helicopter flying time away, would have been primed to come and blow up bridges in order to slow the advance of any enemy ground troops.

One good thing about Hannover was that I became close to Gail, a 25-year-old midwife from Blackpool who became my best friend in the mess. Gail is one of the loveliest, most open and honest people I know – though she can sometimes be almost too honest for her own good, not always thinking things through before speaking. It can be a charming trait, but it was to inadvertently cause me a problem later on.

Not too long into the posting, we were getting along famously; we would discuss anything and everything, very intently, often disagreeing but always respecting one another's opinions. She was great fun to be with. I loved her energy and direct approach to everything.

One evening as we discussed relationships, I was yet again weighing up the pros and cons of telling her my 'secret'. I of course did, and she gave it some thought before rather nervously asking, 'You don't fancy me, do you?' She was clearly embarrassed to ask, and I was at great pains to assure her that no – much as I thought the world of her, I had no romantic or lustful feelings towards her at all. She seemed reassured by this and I thought no more of it. The next time we were quaffing beers in the Ernst August Brauerei she took a long swig, looked at me quizzically and asked, 'Why don't you fancy me? What's wrong with me?'

Looking back, I had a lot of fun in Hannover, and settled in quickly. I was thoroughly enjoying the transition from private to lieutenant and I was incredibly proud to be a QA. It crossed my mind that one or two who whined about the strict regimented way in which things were done tended to be those who seemed either a wee bit lazy or, worse still, had no intention of staying longer than it would take to find a rich doctor or Household Cavalry officer to put a ring on their finger. The vast majority were just fabulous, though – great nurses and fun people with whom to work and spend quality time. Life was good and I had no idea how things were about to change.

I was settling well in Hannover and had been there for six months before an event happened that was to change the course of my life. It was a direct result of alcohol-fuelled impetuosity. I am perhaps going to risk sounding as if I'm offering excuses here, but, in for a penny … A small group of us had spent the evening down in the mess bar. As this was what was known as the public rooms, we were at that time obliged to wear either skirts or dresses after 7.00 pm: trousers were not permitted for the ladies! As it got late and most of the others had gone up to bed, only three of us were left – Gail, my closest friend and confidante, Mags, another ward sister, and me. The conversation turned to a fellow officer, Celia. Mags was telling us that she had been spreading malicious rumours and suggesting that people thought I might be queer. Gail and Mags knew someone who had recently arrived from CMH Aldershot. She had started the rumour mill turning and now Celia apparently felt it was incumbent upon her to bring it to the attention of her fellow officers. Gail was fully aware of my 'pre-existing confusion', so we both laughed it off as stupid gossip and tried to play it down. Mags, however, really had the bit between her teeth, to the point where you would have thought they'd been bad-mouthing her. It was odd and made me wonder if there was more to her response than met the eye; a case of 'methinks the lady doth protest too much'. But I also knew she'd had boyfriends so didn't linger long on that particular musing. We were drinking Grolsch, a fairly potent beer, and enjoying the banter, but Gail decided it was time to turn in. I had always been a night owl and wasn't really ready for bed, and thought she was being a party pooper. To this day, no matter how exhausted I might be, it's still as if a switch clicks in my head at 9.00 pm and … boom: I'm wide awake, raring to go! For this reason I have always preferred night shifts to days.

Mags left about ten to fifteen minutes after Gail, amidst much ribbing about what a wussy wimp she was being. Her parting shot was that I was always welcome to pop in for a natter later, as long as I brought some Grolsch with me (she knew I had just added a six-pack to my bar tab!). She also said that she'd been having difficulty sleeping recently, although it wasn't until later that I found out the reason why. After downing another bottle, I decided to go up. As I mounted the stairs I was inwardly bemoaning the fact that most of my officer friends seemed to be early bird wimps, unlike we Army trained nurses. These direct-entry NHS girls just weren't as much fun; bloody lightweights!

I could see Mags's light was on as I neared her door, so I thought, sod it, and knocked. 'Who is it?' she asked softly, and then said 'Come in', once I said it was me.

The room was in subdued light and she had the soundtrack to *The Rocky Horror Picture Show* playing in the background. Earlier in the evening we'd had a fairly deep and intense discussion about the film and in particular, its open attitude towards sexuality and experimentation. I always loved musicals but it was my best friend from school, Viv, who'd introduced me to this cult hit. Listening to her LP was quite an eye-opener in my youth and we saw one of the earliest stage productions at the Comedy Theatre in London. Mags motioned me to come over and sit beside her on her bed. She was lying under her quilt wearing a T-shirt. I offered her a Grolsch and she laughed before saying, 'Fuck it, why not?'

We sat companionably, listening and then quietly singing along to the songs until that famous refrain – 'Don't dream it, be it' – about being true to who you are, started. There was a palpable tension in the air, and for what felt like many minutes, we kept looking at one another quite intently, then looking away as if embarrassed or afraid of what might happen if we kept staring. Our eyes were scanning one another's features – whizzing from eyes to lips, jawline, hair, back to mouth, tongues nervously licking increasingly dry lips. The moment when we eventually leaned into one another and began to kiss was utterly natural and wholly mutual. Neither of us initiated it – it just happened. I would later discover that her statement of events read very differently to mine, but to my dying day, I can only speak my truth.

She was a good kisser and we spent many minutes freely exploring one another. She snaked one arm around my neck and the other around my waist. My right hand went under her T-shirt and I began to caress her breast. Then she pulled away, looking down and saying, 'God, this is moving too fast for me.' I stopped right away. In the days that followed, things went back to normal. However, after that incident it often felt to me as if Mags was most definitely playing games. On a number of occasions when we were standing in a circle in a noisy bar, I thought she was deliberately moving very close to me, pressing her thigh against my leg and sometimes brushing against me as she leaned across in front of me to retrieve her drinks.

It took me a very long time to fully understand the strange chain of events that led to that moment in August 1987, when my life would be forever changed. Everything leads back to one person who, although not directly involved in my story, had a massive impact upon how I came to find myself accused. She was called Elspeth, and was a friend of Mags and Mel. Elspeth had apparently been a victim of deeply traumatic events when she was a young girl. This had naturally affected her enormously and she was being increasingly troubled by dreadful, vivid and deeply disturbing nightmares as a significant anniversary approached. Mags and Mel were doing their best to help her get through this stressful time but we were becoming steadily more worried about her sometimes erratic behaviour. They would therefore take turns to either sleep on the floor in her room or get her to stay in their rooms so they could comfort and reassure her if she became distressed. Elspeth's heartbreaking trauma was affecting all three of them, and they were becoming exhausted by their efforts to protect her.

Mel and Mags had been really struggling to cover for Elspeth, whose unpredictable behaviour was beginning to be noticed by colleagues at work and in the mess, and they were fearful as to how to help without putting her into a compromising situation. In those days and in that environment, it wasn't possible to just ring in sick. You had to report to sick parade and see the doctor if you felt too unwell to work. There was a stigma about not coping. As they hadn't wanted to report Elspeth to the medical officer for a psychiatric opinion, they fatefully decided to talk to her boss. Major Pam Harold was well liked and respected. She was known for having a good sense of humour and the staff on her ward seemed to be very happy working as part of her team. She was also widely believed to be part of what was known as the Grey Mafia. There were differing opinions as to what this actually meant. Some said it was a generic term for the more old school senior QA officers – career women in it for the long haul. Others felt it referred to some of the deeply closeted senior officers. There was a tacit understanding that many of the older, higher ranking QA officers were ostensibly single, classic 'spinsters of this parish' – wedded to the job. I recall that Pam would often try to feign heterosexuality. For example, if some handsome young subaltern came into the dining room when a group of us were sitting at a table finishing lunch, she would say in a conspiratorial and not so quiet manner, 'Wash that boy and send him to my room!' These comments simply made anyone hearing them feel uncomfortable. That she felt the need to do it resulted in a painful mix of embarrassment, pity and sadness.

After they'd filled her in on the appalling story, Major Harold wondered out loud whether all Elspeth's terrible experiences might make her susceptible towards developing lesbian tendencies! I was told that it was then that Mags said, 'Oh no; if anyone in the mess has lesbian tendencies, then it's Elaine!'

Thirteen very unlucky words – that's really all it took to initiate the process that ended my career.

Pam Harold immediately asked Mags to explain her remark, reminding her that she should be careful about saying such things as they could have potentially serious ramifications. Pam was insistent, and so Mags told her – according to the statement she later made to Warrant Officer Lentman, the Special Investigation Branch (SIB) investigating officer – that she was in bed one evening having had a few drinks in the bar with other mess members and was asleep, and then found herself waking up in bed with me on top of her, kissing her and with my hand up her T-shirt!

Having apparently established that there was possibly a lust-filled, predatory dyke at loose in the mess – a mess full of innocent, resolutely heterosexual, uniformly irresistible young women (yeah, right!) – Pam felt compelled to take action. So she reported the allegations to Matron, one of the most strait-laced, pious, unsmiling, serious 'Christian' women ever, and it was something that I would face the consequences of in the weeks and months ahead.

I was on a two-five or split shift, working on the families ward. I was in charge that day, Friday, 21 August 1987, because the Captain was away on leave.

Everything was running smoothly, as always; we had a good team who all knew what they were doing and could be relied upon to get on with it.

I was working on the rota in the sister's office when the telephone rang. I heard Matron's cold, clipped tones in the receiver: 'Lieutenant Chambers, I need you to come to my office immediately.' I began to say that it would leave no cover, but she was very curt. 'That doesn't matter. Come straight away.'

I knocked and then went in. I genuinely hadn't the foggiest idea why she wanted to see me so urgently. It even crossed my mind that something dreadful had happened at home with my brother. My brother's alcoholism was getting worse by the day and he had previously attempted suicide. But I was soon sitting stunned to hear what she had to say. She started by asking if I knew why I was here. Of course I didn't, so she told me, wearing a deeply pained and disgusted expression on her face. 'It has come to my attention that you have made unwanted advances to two of your fellow officers. What have you got to say for yourself?'

I felt myself blushing beetroot and could feel the blood pumping in my neck. I just couldn't believe what I was hearing! I tried to calm my pounding heart, taking a deep breath and frantically attempting to compute things. I said that it absolutely wasn't true and that I was totally shocked by what she was saying. I then asked her which officers and what exactly they had said, but she refused to tell me, saying that she had to speak to me first before deciding what course of action to take. Although I knew I had undoubtedly broken military law, I also knew that I most certainly hadn't assaulted anyone. Christ! My technique might well leave a lot to be desired, but I felt what happened had been mutually consensual, and as far as I was concerned, Mel had been the instigator in the first incident.

My mind was reeling …

'So, are you denying the allegations, Lieutenant Chambers?'

'Yes, of course I am. It's absolutely not true.'

'Well, I'm afraid there will have to be an investigation. You are dismissed.'

I returned to the ward and must have looked as if I'd seen a ghost. The staff on duty looked worried. 'Are you alright?' 'You look a bit pale.' 'What did the old cow want?'

Of course I couldn't tell them, so I fobbed them off, and as it was nearly one o'clock, went straight to my room in the mess.

I knew I didn't have long to gather together any evidence that would prove anything at all to do with homosexuality. Time was of the essence, but more importantly, where would I put it? There was no way I could destroy stuff other than by burning it, and there was no access to a shredder, so I thought my best bet would be to hide anything that might be in even the slightest way incriminatory. I started frantically filling two carrier bags with items that might be deemed as fitting the sapphic bill: my diaries, letters, one or two books, a newsletter from the Golden Wheel Lesbian Dating Agency, along with a couple of letters I'd received in Aldershot from other subscribers. I was no longer on their list at the time, so why on earth had I kept them?

It was by now the middle of a Friday afternoon. I had made the fatal mistake of thinking any investigation involving the Royal Military Police Special Investigation Branch wouldn't start before Monday; they were based quite some miles away and it was POETS day (Piss Off Early, Tomorrow's Saturday), so I left the bags on my bed and went round to see if Gail was in. She was also on a split shift that day but had gone into town, probably to meet her young civilian boyfriend, Kai. The only other person I would have trusted, Nessa, was away on annual leave. I toyed with the idea of seeing if I could put the bags in the attic but decided against it because being the afternoon, there were too many people around and I was likely to attract attention if I was seen acting suspiciously. It was a very small hospital of only five wards and an even smaller mixed mess. So I thought I'd catch Gail later, and went back to work.

Just half an hour into the second part of the shift, Matron rang and told me to come to her office. Once again, I had to tell my staff I had to go to see Matron and leave the ward without RGN cover, but without telling them why, everyone would soon be jumping to wild conclusions. This time, as I entered her office she wasn't alone. A stocky man, probably in his forties, and a very young looking woman, perhaps in her early twenties, were standing by her impressive desk. My heart sank. Goddammit! To me, their number two dress uniforms gave no clue, but their bright red forage caps did: Military Police. Didn't these people have homes to go to?

Introductions were made, all very charming and polite, then the allegations were repeated and I was asked if I had anything I'd like to say. I was advised that I wasn't being charged with anything at this stage, merely that they needed to know what my response was. Once again, I refuted the allegations most vehemently. This time I was told the names of my accusers: Captain Melanie Benn and Lieutenant Margaret Taft. I was then given a brief outline of what they were saying had happened. Because I instantly knew my career was at an end, right at that very moment, I understood as clearly as anything that I was now fighting to defend my reputation in order to avoid being punished for an offence I had *not* committed. So I looked WO2 Lentman in the eye and told him in a firm and steady voice that I was being painted as some kind of heavy-handed dyke (Matron visibly flinched) and that it was simply not true, and that I hadn't assaulted anyone. I felt overwhelmed by the adrenalin borne of a potent mix of fear, anger and indignation.

He then advised me that, due to my denying the allegations, he would have to carry out an official investigation. He said that because of the lateness of the hour, he would leave the questioning until after the weekend. I breathed a sigh of relief. 'But,' he said, 'I would like to go your room in order to conduct a search of your personal effects.' Oh my god! The image of two full bags of 'evidence' sitting waiting on my bed almost caused me to laugh out loud. I was frantically trying to think of some sort of stalling tactic. I told him my room key was in my bag back in the ward office and I was hoping I might be able to say it was bit of a mess. 'Will you give me five minutes and I'll meet you there?' Another barmy notion, given that I'd been the fastest runner at basic fitness training, was to race ahead to my room and throw the bags out of the window. Before I could give voice to any such crazed thoughts, he said, 'That's fine. We'll come with you.'

Everyone saw me get my handbag from the office, accompanied by two Red Caps and Matron – what on earth they thought at that moment I'll never know, but some of the rumours that later surfaced were nothing short of hilarious. Gail told me about them: I'd stolen controlled drugs; I was a drug addict; I'd stolen petty cash from the mess bar; I'd somehow fiddled my expenses or mess bills; I'd had an affair with a senior married male officer.

Not one of these was remotely near the truth, so a few weeks into the subsequent investigation, I asked everyone I worked with on the ward to meet in the ward kitchen. Even though WO2 Lentman had made it very clear that I shouldn't talk about the case to anyone, I knew I'd be leaving the Army when it was over, and I was determined that such ludicrous rumours were going to be dispelled.

So without going into all the details, I basically told them the essential stuff, which to my mind was the fact that they had enough evidence to prove that I had previously had liaisons with women. Not one member of staff was bothered by this. In fact, if anything, it led to me having more support. I was given beautiful bouquets with lovely messages, and cards were sent from across the ranks and in the mess.

Nearly everyone who showed me such immense kindness professed their shock at the stupidity of the ban. The vast majority of my colleagues were heterosexual and were the very personnel the high ranking officers constantly claimed would 'leave in protest' if openly gay people were allowed to serve alongside them. These patronising proclamations, which assumed that the rank-and-file servicemen or servicewomen held the same archaic, irrational homophobic beliefs as those who voiced them, were utterly offensive and presumptuous. I experienced none of the reactions that were cited with regular, predictable monotony over the subsequent years of battle against such ignorant bigotry.

When I re-read my diaries after they were given back to me in January 1988 – nearly six months after they were bagged up as exhibits – I was quite surprised to realise how terribly tormented I had felt while battling to accept my sexuality. The diaries had finally been sent back to me at home in Harrow Weald after I had returned to Civvy Street, delivered personally by two men who I presume would have been Royal Military policemen in plain clothes. I didn't enquire, nor invite them in for a cuppa. I felt a need to exorcise the mental image that had manifested itself in my mind – gruff, blokey SIB officers laughing themselves stupid at my most intimate yearnings and pinings, right back to early adolescence. They had taken all of my diaries, even those predating my joining the forces by many years. What possible relevance could they have had to present-day accusations of assault? Did they truly believe that there would be some pertinent evidence to support my detractors' bullshit? That I would have taken great delight in writing a blow-by-blow account of how aroused and powerful I felt as I allegedly ravished these poor defenceless women against their will? Luckily I hadn't recorded any of the details about my first truly revelatory lesbian experience with Sadie. Sure, there was mention of vaguely erotic dreams I'd had about my unrequited crushes, along with some fairly lame non-sexual poetry, but nothing solid enough for them to extend their sordid witch-hunt. However, sadly, the letters I had kept had led them straight to their target.

My first interrogation took place on Monday, 24 August 1987. The late 1980s was a time of technical innovations such as CD players, mobile phones, Walkmans and the like, so imagine my shock when I realised that there was no equipment to record the interview! Whilst that may sound archaically funny, in reality, it was incredibly annoying and frustrating. WO2 Lentman would pose a question and then expect me to answer slowly … enough … to … let … him … write … it … down … in … longhand! When one is attempting to prove one's innocence in relation to allegations of indecent assault and give an account of what happened, this is just ludicrous, because the train of thought gets well and truly lost while waiting for the scribe to catch up. He wasn't even able to write shorthand. I was totally gobsmacked. It also made the whole process hellishly laborious and time-consuming. I cannot help but imagine it was a deliberate ploy of the SIB, designed specifically to wear people down.

I had been falsely accused of indecent assault against a female aged 16 or over, and of making advances of a sexual nature, neither of which were offences exclusively nor solely applicable to a military environment. Offences tried in military courts can also be brought to civilian courts. I fully understood the devastating seriousness of the allegations, and I was absolutely terrified of this and believed it was a possibility. This unbearable prospect had been explained to me over the telephone by my legal counsel. I'd asked as many questions as I could think of. But my head was all over the place – a complete maelstrom of chaotic thoughts crashing around. How much I really retained or even understood is a moot point.

So I complied, to the letter, giving as detailed an account as I possibly could of what had occurred. Although the allegations had completely flummoxed and mystified me, the one thing that kept me going throughout the entire time was the knowledge that I knew I was telling the whole truth – despite the mortal embarrassment of having to do so … very … slowly … so that Warrant Officer Lentman could write it all down!

My honesty was to cost me dear. In hindsight, I'm stunned at my complete stupidity, but can only put it down to the fear and my inexperience. I really believed I was being questioned purely to establish whether or not there would be any hard evidence to convert mere allegations into full-blown, answerable in court, conviction-carrying charges. I therefore concentrated on doing exactly as I had been advised.

As the process continued, I came to realise I had totally fucked everything up and was desperate to get to the phone to ring Sadie and warn her. And of course, that's exactly what I did. Sadie was naturally completely incensed at how bloody stupid I was; she even went as far as to ask if I'd deliberately dropped her in it as some sort of revenge! I pleaded with her, trying desperately to explain how hard it was being questioned in this stilted, stop-start fashion, unable to really get to grips with what I wanted to say. She wasn't interested and seemed very concerned that I hadn't mentioned the name of her last long-term female relationship prior to having got married. I assured her truthfully that, no, I absolutely never mentioned the woman with whom she had been involved. I later heard that as a result of my words, two SIB officers arrived at her married quarters. I suppose she was prepared for them, thanks to my phone call. Although they apparently searched the entire flat from top to bottom, nothing was found that could be bagged and tagged.

I only spoke to Sadie once more after that fateful call and mistakenly believed for many years that she too would have been forced to leave the corps after admitting that we had been involved. She had been shown part of my statement by the SIB, the legality of which (showing my statement I mean) I was unsure about even then.

Later I was told that Sadie had in fact, at great risk to herself, corroborated my story about our brief 'affair'. In one way, Sadie's statement should have been supportive of my version of events, but alas, WO2 Lentman saw it differently. When I was next summoned to see him he tore a strip off me. I was quite shocked at his vehemence and found myself blushing profusely as he berated me for jeopardising everything. Didn't I realise I could be charged with deliberately suborning witnesses? I'd never even heard of that word before.

In any case, Sadie had told Lentman that she knew I had been accused of indecent assault but also that she knew I hadn't done it. When he asked how she knew, she said, 'She's not that kind of person; she's too nice. She's afraid of rejection, she couldn't indecently assault anybody.'

During the first week or two of the investigation, as Lentman began extending his enquiries elsewhere, I was in a chaotic state of shock, my mind frantically trying to make sense of what had happened. I just could not understand why, if Mel and Mags had genuinely felt so repulsed by what had happened, they had continued to interact with me, socialise with me and treat me as a friend. None of it made any sense. I went over and over things in my head, trying to figure out why, and scribbling notes in a little book. I was desperate to find anything that might help prove that I was the only one telling the truth. My friends and colleagues were amazingly supportive and I somehow kept going. Only my closest friends knew more about what was going on. Others would have heard plenty of rumours and supposition through the usual gossipy grapevine. And I had no idea what my accusers were telling my friends; I could only hope that the nature of the accusations might be a little too embarrassing for them to freely share with anyone endeavouring to find out, but the stress of not knowing what was happening behind the scenes was really getting to me.

When things had first kicked off, I had known I would, at some point, probably sooner rather than later, need to go home to my parents. I knew I would have to tell them. It being such a long-winded and convoluted story, I realised it would be impossible to try to telephone them and talk them through it. I would never gather enough 5 Deutschmark coins, and there was no guarantee of privacy as the phone was stuck on a wall in a corridor of the mess. I had therefore written a very long letter, which ran to twenty-one double sides of A5 Basildon Bond, because I really felt I needed to try to fully explain the background to what had happened. After posting it, I was sick with worry – what if they disowned me or were so ashamed and disappointed in me that they didn't want me home? Or, worse still, what if they bought into the whole 'no smoke without fire' notion? I was beside myself with anxiety, yet was still expected to work through the whole process on my own. It was testament to my wonderful parents that I was welcomed home with open arms.

As the investigation lumbered slowly on, I began to feel calmer. I worked as hard as I could and felt supported by all those around me. But the days drew on and it would be some time before my anxiety was finally put to rest …

I will never know what happened to make Mel decide to come clean on 9 September 1987, but thank God she did. I only got to read what she eventually admitted to some ten years later, after acquiring the information from the Ministry of Defence under the Freedom of Information Act:

> I kept thinking back on my incident with Lieutenant Chambers and almost convinced myself that something very bad had been pushed on me. In my haste and in trying to protect myself in case anyone thought I was lesbian, the facts from my previous statement were given. These being untrue. I never said to Major Harold at this point that Elaine Chambers had assaulted me. Following this statement, I wish to put into writing that I never realised the outcome of what my lies would be. I now realise to the full and deeply regret what I have done.

She was reported for alleged unnatural conduct, and for allegedly attempting to pervert the course of justice. These things too I only discovered ten years after the events. Amongst the pain of reliving such awful times by reading these documents, there were also beautiful nuggets of love, support and protection – ultimately heartbreaking in so many ways, but testament to the humanity we share in the Armed Forces, despite our differences and our travails. Although I was terribly sad about what happened to her, Mel's action in coming clean really was vitally important to me, saving me from a much more damning and potentially life-threatening outcome. I truly believe that there would have been a distinct possibility of my committing suicide if I had faced trial and been found guilty of such a disgusting offence. Although Mel's admission was of course incredibly useful to me, it transpired that the SIB were prepared to invest even more of their resources in the investigation as they extended the witch-hunt and looked for new scalps.

In my life since these events, I have tried to focus on being positive and upbeat. Admittedly, I have not always succeeded, but for the most part, I've done alright: living a life of mindfulness, and living in the moment, relishing anything and everything good that comes my way. One of my all-time favourite quotes comes

Our first London Pride, 1991. The banner I made was not welcomed by the community!

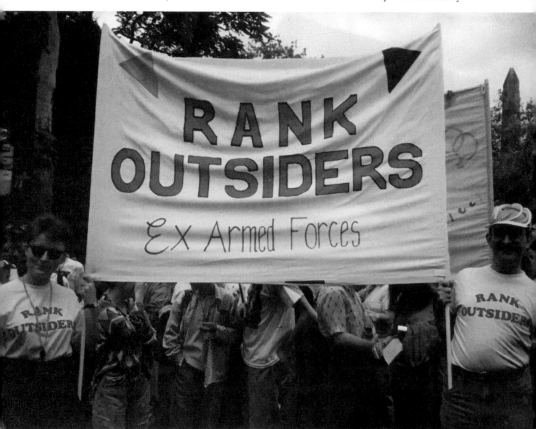

from the incredible James Dean, my number one idol: 'Dream as if you'll live forever – live as if you'll die today.'

So that's what I do now, no matter what misfortune comes my way. I refuse to allow myself to stay down for too long – life being, as a well-worn cliché rightly says, way too short. I relish those moments of sheer joy; they lift my spirits to a point where I almost feel as if I could levitate and float just an inch or two above the ground, unseen by those around me, but truly aware that one day I might fly high. So I live for those fleeting moments, those delicious oases of unfettered sublime happiness and delight. Until the next one comes along, this 'queer angel' will be patiently waiting, now looking forward, not back.

Extracts adapted from *This Queer Angel* by
Elaine Chambers (Unbound, 2019)

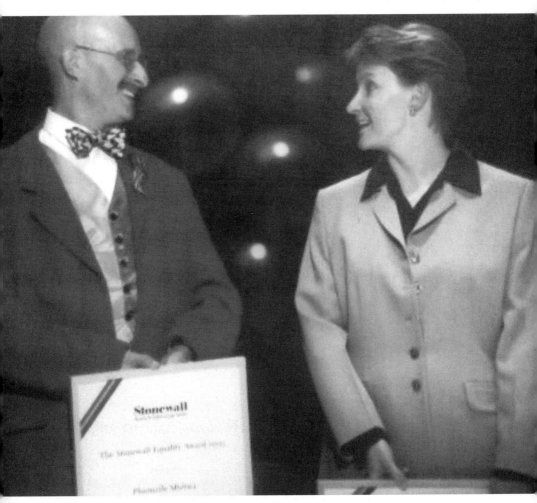

Robert Ely and me presenting the Stonewall awards at the Royal Albert Hall, 1994.

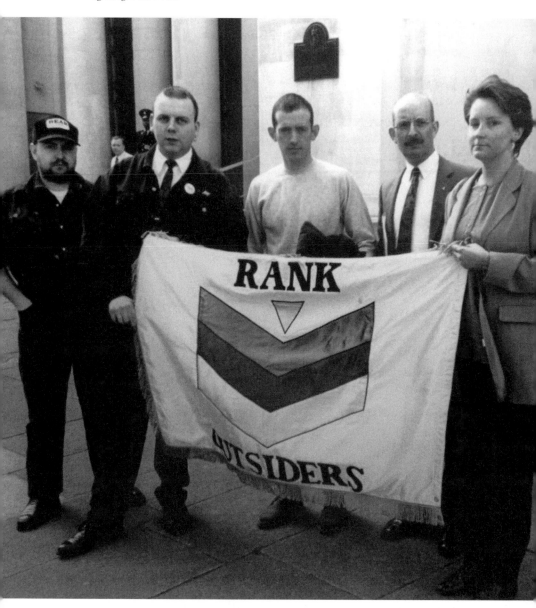

Being moved along by security outside the MoD, 1995. Left to right: Ricky Gellison, Mike Sansom, Robert Ely and me.

Chapter 8

Sea Change: From Closet to Pride
Commander Roly Woods
Royal Navy

I joined the Royal Navy by steam train – no, I'm not so old that I remember the golden age of steam; it was actually the Dart Valley steam train from Paignton to Dartmouth, but some aspects of naval life in the late 1970s and 1980s did still bear a very strong resemblance to that Victorian era:

> It was illegal to be gay in the military.

> You would receive a dishonourable discharge if discovered to be gay, which meant it would be almost impossible to get regular employment in Civvy Street.

> We were regularly lectured on the wrongs of being gay, including the negative impact on team cohesion and operational effectiveness – an argument that was used right up until the ECHR judgment in 1999.

> Homosexuals were classed as a threat to security because of the risk of blackmail by hostile intelligence services (which neatly ignored the fact that we were only blackmailable because the system said it was wrong to be gay!).

So why did I want to join such a bigoted organisation? Surely there were better career options? Well, I fancied the excitement and adventure of the Royal Navy, travelling the world and avoiding the dreaded office 9 to 5. As a late developer I didn't come out to myself until my late twenties, which was probably a reflection of both military life and wider societal issues of the 1970s and 1980s, and I had had several fulfilling relationships with women in my twenties. By the time I acknowledged my sexuality, I was enjoying a successful naval career. I had had early command of an RN ship and was a poster boy for the RN as the youngest CO at sea – the strapline was 'Your Own Company at 27' – and I really wanted to realise my full potential in a job I loved doing.

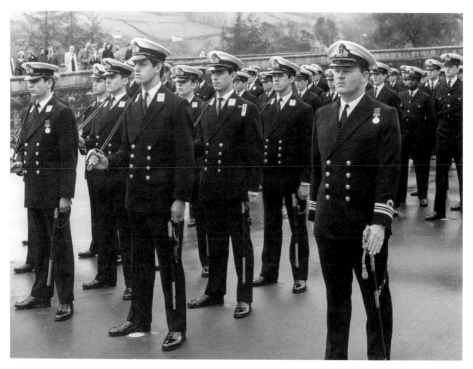

Midshipman Woods on parade at Britannia Royal Naval College Dartmouth (front centre, with HRH Prince Andrew a footstep behind).

Having experimented and subsequently taken the plunge into a closeted gay life, the highs and lows were soon apparent. In the 1980s, the only gay bar in my then home town of Exeter was the infamous Acorn. A somewhat unprepossessing bar in the middle of a dreary roundabout in the city centre, it was the focal point of gay life in Exeter at the time. Determined but petrified, one Saturday evening I headed out, dressed in what I thought would be acceptable in a gay bar: tight jeans and a granddad shirt, which was in fact a naval officer's shirt, described on the label as 'shirt, white, collar detached, officer's'. I employed my best counter-intelligence techniques on my way there, taking a circuitous route, doubling back, stopping to look at reflections in shop windows and looking over my shoulder to ensure I was not being followed. Sounds paranoid and melodramatic now, I know, but that was a standard feeling for many years whenever I ventured out to a new gay venue, either in the UK or when deployed abroad. Heart seriously pounding, I walked into the Acorn and discovered a whole new world – it was rammed with an all-male crowd of all ages, pumping music and, for me, a very exciting vibe. Very self-conscious and in urgent need of Dutch courage, I ordered a pint, found a corner where I could see the door, with half an eye on how to extract myself if I met anyone I knew, and gradually started to relax. As a newbie I was the object of interest and was soon chatting,

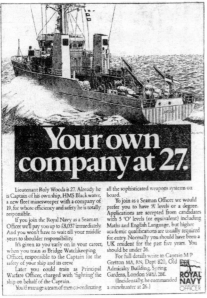

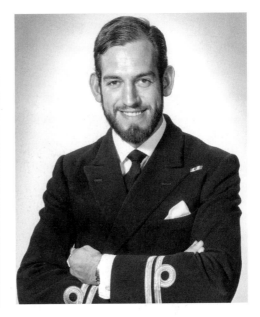

Under the recruitment image:

Lieutenant Roly Woods is 27. Already he is Captain of his own ship, HMS Blackwater, a new fleet minesweeper with a company of 19, for whose efficiency and safety he is totally responsible.

If you join the Royal Navy as a Seaman Officer we'll pay you up to £8,037 immediately. And you won't have to wait till your middle years to shoulder responsibility.

It's given to you early on in your career, when you train as Bridge Watchkeeping Officer, responsible to the Captain for the safety of your ship and its crew.

Later you could train as Principal Warfare Officer, charged with 'fighting' the ship on behalf of the Captain.

You'd manage a team of men co-ordinating all the sophisticated weapons systems on board.

To join as a Seaman Officer we would prefer you to have 'A' levels or a degree. Applications are accepted from candidates with 5 'O' levels (or equivalent) including Maths and English Language, but higher academic qualifications are usually required for entry. Normally you should have been a UK resident for the past five years. You should be under 26.

For full details write to Captain M P Gretton MA, RN, Dept 820, Old Admiralty Building, Spring Gardens, London SW1A 2BE.

(Incidentally, he commanded a minehunter at 26.)

ROYAL NAVY OFFICER

Above left and right: Lieutenant Roly Woods, 'Your own company at 27' – RN recruitment campaign, 1986.

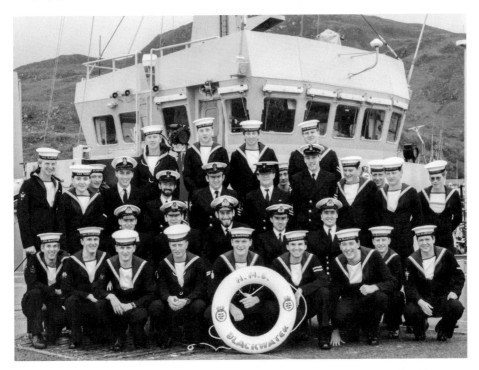

Commanding Officer HMS *Blackwater* on Fishery Protection duties, 1986, pictured amidst a team I was extremely proud to command.

again self-consciously and with a partial cover story about who I was and what I did. That first evening passed in a flash.

Very early on, following my first foray into the gay subculture of Exeter, I met my first long-term partner, Peter. We met at the Acorn when I gallantly rescued him from the unwelcome attention of an apparent competitor. Good-looking, 6'4", 22, slim and extrovert, wearing very skimpy tight blue shorts, he was exciting, passionate and FUN – everything that I was looking for. He and I quickly hit it off and I was soon head over heels in love. Working away from home in the week, I experienced the well-known emotional rollercoaster of the weekend commuter – rushing home from a very intense, year-long, warfare training course in Portsmouth, cursing the Friday traffic, to enjoy a passionate weekend with my partner, and then having to wrench myself away on a Sunday evening or very early on a Monday morning to return to base in Portsmouth. Whilst the weekend commute is common to thousands of people, the huge difference for me was that I was unable to be open with my close friends and colleagues at work. I had to fabricate a completely separate lifestyle of girlfriends and straight nights out and was unable to share the highs and lows that I was experiencing with my closest and most trusted friends. This presented a huge dichotomy, which affected how I lived my life, and there are echoes of it even today. I'm still a very private, some would say secretive, person and it takes time for me to be fully open with people. This hidden part of my life continued for many years – later in my career, when returning from eight-month RN deployments, Peter would come on board with family friends to disguise the nature of his relationship with me, and we could only watch as loved ones hugged passionately on the jetty or in the wardroom. We had to save our hugs for more private moments once we were at home on leave. This conflict was further complicated because I was sharing my Exeter city-centre, Victorian town house with my mother, Alice, who ran it as a guest house while I was away at sea or on courses. Needless to say, I wasn't out to my family at that stage, but in spite of all this, I had a great relationship with them in what was effectively a 'don't ask, don't tell' scenario. Fortunately, Peter and my mum got on like a house on fire and no questions were asked. In fact, they're still great buddies today.

Peter and I had 'separate' rooms on a common landing in our end of terrace townhouse, which, give or take a noisy floorboard, worked out pretty well. An outgoing, sociable guy, Peter had a wide circle of friends in Exeter's small gay community, and they welcomed me with open arms. In spite of this, however, I remained very cautious, even paranoid. I would always introduce myself as a merchant navy officer and, because I have a distinctive first name, I used my middle name of Phil when introducing myself to anybody in gay circles. My rationale for doing so was to give a degree of plausible deniability should anyone from my military life bump into me with my gay friends and I could claim confusion/mis-identity. This would not have been a strong defence but it gives an idea of the way I had to think and behave at the time. There was certainly lots of scope for confusion, and even today, some thirty years later, Peter's family and friends from that era still call me Phil when our paths occasionally cross.

Life became even more complicated when buddies from my various ships came to visit, either for a meal before a 'straight' night on the town in Exeter or for a whole weekend. You can imagine the careful choreography that was required to ensure that my gay friends didn't bump into my straight friends, and vice versa. Who was going to be where and when? I had a straight pub crawl, which carefully avoided the bars frequented by my gay friends, that I used whenever the Navy was in town and when I didn't have to hide behind this façade, Peter and I would meet up with the gay gang wherever the fun was that night. This all worked surprisingly well, all things considered, and Peter was a complete star. In hindsight, it did cause additional stress and unnecessary emotional strain, but that said, for all my apparent paranoia and concerns, we actually had a great time and our spacious lounge was the scene of many a late-night gathering of our different social groups.

Having qualified as a Principal Warfare Officer (PWO), the officer who advises the Captain on how best to employ his weapons to best effect in a tactical, war-fighting situation, I joined one of the most up-to-date and senior ships in the Royal Navy at the time – HMS *Cornwall*. She was a newly built, Batch 3 Type 22 frigate with a senior RN captain in command and I was soon deploying to exotic locations, flying the flag and putting my newly learned war-fighting skills into practice in complex naval exercises with various allies.

As a PWO I was fortunate enough to have my own cabin on board. It was sparse but pretty comfortable by naval standards: a small desk to work at, work chair, sink with a folding cover, white shatterproof wardrobes with a couple of shoe drawers underneath, and a fold-down bunk, just about long enough for my 6'2" frame, covered with the standard MoD chintz covers of questionable taste and a bottle green carpet. The total floor area was probably 2.5 metres by 2 metres and, of course, the ubiquitous trunking for cables and pipes ran through the middle of it. You quickly became accustomed to the permanent background hiss of the air conditioning, not really noticing it, even though it seems very loud when you first hear it. Indeed, if it ever stopped, you immediately paid attention because stopping the ventilation system was, and still is, a standard immediate response to a fire on board, in order to stop the spread of smoke; if your cabin went quiet as the air conditioning crash-stopped, you paid attention.

So, I had my own space – compact and functional but private, which was a definite plus. Oh, and as a PWO, I also had my own safe for keeping classified documents in. Clearly this was essential for keeping classified material secure, but conveniently it also allowed me to keep extracts from the *Spartacus Gay Travel Guide* away from prying eyes and thus my private life as secure as national secrets!

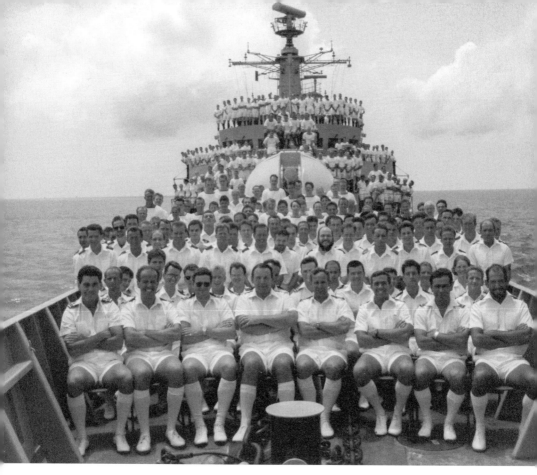

Lieutenant Commander Roly Woods, Principal Warfare Officer HMS *Cornwall* (front row, right) in the Caribbean in 1992 on duty as the West Indies Guard Ship.

The *Spartacus* guide was an essential element for making full use of my limited free time ashore in foreign ports.

HMS *Cornwall* deployed to the Caribbean as the West Indies Guard Ship (WIGS) in the early 1990s. Her Majesty's Government (HMG) maintains a ship in the Caribbean during the hurricane season to provide immediate Humanitarian Assistance and Disaster Relief (HADR) support to the Overseas Territories (OTs) in the event of a major hurricane. Of course, when not required for HADR operations, the ship flies the flag on defence engagement duties, visiting the OTs, conducting counternarcotics (CN) operations and exercising with allies in the region, including the United States Navy (USN). While not quite the four days in port, followed by one day at sea to recover before the next round of cocktail parties of yesteryear, *Cornwall*'s programme wasn't too shabby. We would spend a few weeks at sea conducting various naval war games, training missile firings and suchlike before heading in for our next port visit. Following a useful and very sociable briefing weekend at the US Navy HQ in Key West over spring break weekend, we arrived in Pensacola, Florida, for a two-week maintenance period.

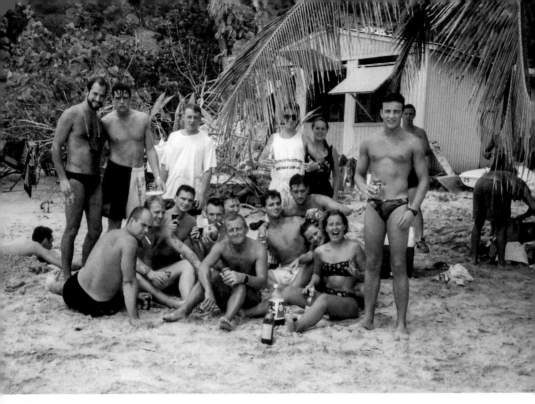

HMS *Cornwall* Caribbean deployment, 1992 – divisional banyan (barbeque) after much hard work on patrol.

My extract from the *Spartacus* gay travel guide quickly came into its own and I was soon making friends in the local gay bar – The Roundup. Pensacola is a relatively small town so I had to employ my usual counter-intelligence techniques – scouting the location, checking for anyone from the ship's company in the vicinity, excuse at the ready should there be anyone from the ship in there when I entered and also in case anyone came in by mistake while I was there. This, of course, was fine initially but became more challenging once I'd been there a couple of times and got to know the locals and the bar staff; it was obvious pretty quickly that the visiting Brit was from the large grey RN warship down the road. As it happened, the gods were smiling on me. I was chatting to my sailors on board at stand easy one forenoon during the visit and heard all about the exploits of Ginge – a very red-headed Scouser who was one of my very straight able seaman gunners. Apparently the worse for wear after an afternoon's drinking in Pensacola, he couldn't find his way back to the ship. Using his initiative, he headed to the nearest bar to ask for directions, whereupon he was welcomed with open arms and didn't have to buy a drink for the rest of the night. You guessed – he'd found The Roundup! He was proudly telling his dit of free drinks and friendly locals to all and sundry on board, including me, as his divisional officer (DO). Fortunately, I had been the duty officer on board at the time he was enjoying the delights of The Roundup and so had not been in my usual seat at the bar, where I'd been for most nights that week. Phew! Needless to say, I was a tad more cautious around The Roundup for the rest of the visit in case anyone thought about following in Ginge's footsteps for free 'wets' … but I also had to go back and thank the boys for not letting on to Ginge that one of his shipmates was a new regular at the bar!

A new joiner to the wardroom during the deployment was Craig Jones. He chose a great time to join: alongside in Bermuda at the start of the deployment. He managed to avoid months of sea trials, and the full range of demanding operational sea training (OST), during which the ship is prepared for all eventualities, from all-out warfare and onboard emergencies to HADR ops. This is an intense time, hard work and very wearing, but also very satisfying, great for team building, and on completion, the ship is ready for anything. Craig managed to avoid the rigours of OST and a stormy Atlantic crossing, arriving on board for the first cocktail party in Bermuda and the rest of the Caribbean deployment! He and I got on very well from day one and became firm friends – a subconscious gay affinity between two closeted gay RN officers perhaps, as we certainly weren't out to each other then – and it's a friendship that endures to this day. We would regularly hang out together and had similar interests, and we each had large divisions of sailors for

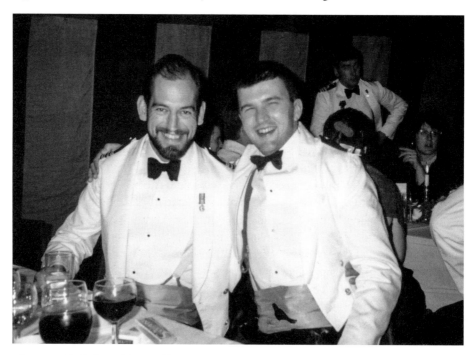

Lieutenant Craig Jones joins HMS *Cornwall* just in time for the fun in Bermuda. The bird on our cummerbunds is the Cornish chough and their gold colour represents the 15 Cornish bezants in the Duchy of Cornwall's heraldic crest.

whom we were responsible. Numerous runs ashore followed throughout our time on board together, both in the Caribbean and the Far East, where we deployed the following year. During time back in our home port of Devonport, Craig would come to stay with me in Exeter for the occasional weekend to escape the ship and I would take him to my usual straight haunts. He got on well with Peter, although we were still very circumspect and discreet.

Shortly after leaving HMS *Cornwall*, Craig again came to stay in Exeter for the weekend. Another good night out followed, visiting some of the great straight pubs in the city centre. Against my better judgment, my partner Peter persuaded us to go upstairs from one of the pubs to The Loft – the only gay nightclub in Exeter. Several of Peter's and my friends were there and we had a quick drink before I became sufficiently uncomfortable about the risk of being outed and we left. When we got back, Peter went to bed while Craig and I stayed up, putting the world to rights over a nightcap, as was our habit. Then came the big reveal – not from me to Craig, but from Craig to me! He told me he was gay, that the girlfriend he often spoke about was imaginary, and that was that! I immediately told him that I was gay too, and that Peter was my partner. Needless to say, he wasn't completely surprised! Thus our friendship developed as we exchanged stories and frustrations and laughed over our exploits in HMS *Cornwall* – we realised that we must be the only gay guys ever to go to Bangkok and have an entirely straight visit there!

Craig and Peter were already good friends and Craig now became a regular fixture on the Exeter scene. We introduced him to the Exeter gang, which included a charming teenager by the name of Adam. Craig and Adam were soon very close friends and it was a good match – they're still together today some twenty-four years later!

Another incident that stands out from that era and reflects the challenges of the time followed a late-night chat over a coffee in my cabin with a junior rating during one deployment. It was a Saturday at sea in the Indian Ocean, the weather was great and there had been a barbecue on the flight deck under the stars for the whole ship's company, accompanied by the authorised couple of tins of beer. Towards the end of the evening, I got chatting with Geordie, a normally cheerful stoker who was clearly a bit down. It was soon clear that he had been having problems with his girlfriend. After talking for some time, it was becoming chilly on the upper deck and we went to my cabin to continue our conversation. He was appreciative of my support and we had a great chat, touching on many issues. Sometime later, he returned to his mess deck in a much better frame of mind and I turned in. First thing next morning, I was summoned to the Executive Officer's (XO) cabin and was interrogated about my late-night private meeting with a junior rating in my cabin. This took me completely by surprise, after what had been an entirely innocent and constructive conversation. I protested my innocence and voiced my surprise at the intimation that I had behaved improperly. The XO took my explanation at face value and no more was said, although I subsequently discovered that the sailor had also been interrogated by the Master-at-Arms, the ship's onboard policeman, as to what had happened in my cabin. Of course nothing untoward had happened and that was the end of the incident, but it was an uncomfortable and unnecessary experience that reflected the mores of the time.

People often ask why I didn't come out to my family much earlier than I actually did. For the record, I came out to my older brother Andy some time before I did to my mother. Andy's always been there for me, especially in times of crisis, and has been a rock whenever I have needed him. He was entirely unfazed that I was gay and was full of sensible advice. He respected my decision not to tell my mum just yet but didn't think she would be too upset. I finally came out to her as I was sadly splitting up from Peter. By this time he was living in my Exeter house full-time with my mum and I wanted her to know what was going on in case things got messy. So I took her for a drink at the White Hart Inn in the city. Over large G&Ts, I explained that Peter and I were more than just good friends and that we were going our separate ways. Unsurprisingly, Mum was not taken aback or even surprised, and was more concerned for my happiness than over my being gay. She recognised the challenges that being gay posed for my naval career but took everything in her stride. Fortunately, although separating from Peter was painful for both of us, we managed it in a mature way and I'm delighted to say we are still firm friends twenty-three years later – in fact, Mum and I attended his wedding to Gary, his great partner of many years, in 2018.

So why didn't I come out earlier to my mum? I think it was a combination of a degree of embarrassment and wanting to protect her. It was the 1970s, and the only gay role models I can recall from the era were the very camp Jon Inman character in *Are You Being Served* and the equally camp Larry Grayson, with his catchphrase 'Shut that door!'. I also wanted to avoid causing any potential hurt or distress. In spring 1982, while serving in the patrol ship HMS *Leeds Castle*, we were directed to sail almost immediately for the Falkland Islands to join the task group there, fighting to retake the islands from the Argentine military, who had seized them a few weeks before. We were all granted twenty-four hours' leave to say goodbye to family and friends and I have a searing memory of my mum crying on the front doorstep of the three-bedroomed semi in Leicester in which I'd grown up. It was one of the few times I'd seen her cry and, on reflection, having lost Michael, one of her three sons, killed a couple of years earlier by a negligent driver in a road traffic accident, she was no doubt petrified of losing another one. I suspect that, subconsciously, this also contributed to my wanting to protect her from hurt and worry, hence not coming out earlier.

A moment of reflection after the Falkland Islands had been recaptured. Paying respects at the grave of Colonel H. Jones VC OBE.

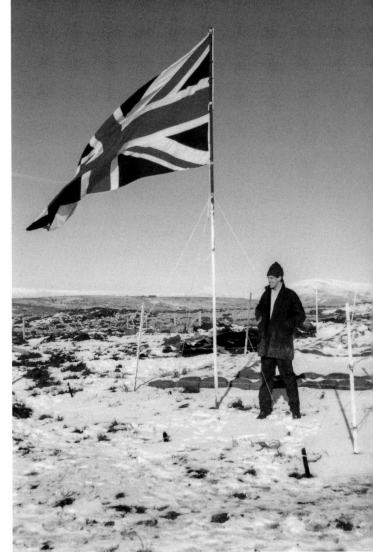

Following a high-speed transit 8,000 miles south, *QE2*, assisted by HMS *Leeds Castle*, transfers her embarked troops for the main assault in San Carlos Water.

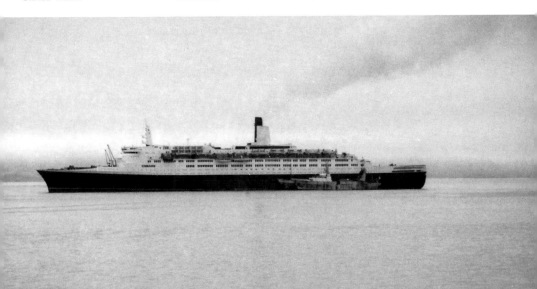

From early on in my naval career, the perils associated with being gay in the military were made very clear. From new entry training onwards, everyone in the military is required to attend an annual security lecture, to ensure the security threats to the military are understood by all. Bear in mind that when I joined we were still in the depths of the Cold War, and the perils of espionage were a major theme of these security briefings. Real-life spying case studies were covered in detail, with a major focus on gay men who were blackmailed into spying for the USSR. Because homosexuality was banned in the military, gay individuals in the forces were susceptible to blackmail, and this issue was heavily emphasised at every security lecture. It seemed obvious to me that if there wasn't a ban in place then there would be no grounds for blackmail – needless to say, I didn't raise this obvious flaw in the security argument, preferring not to draw attention to myself.

Thus, having apparently established that being gay in the military was wrong, it was clearly necessary to make sure that officers were able to identify homosexuals so that they could be rooted out of the military. The regulations were clear, and so a whole cadre of very conservative, mainly entitled and largely unimaginative straight instructors, who were obviously uncomfortable with the subject but who saw it as their duty to ensure the military was purged of this gay menace, very helpfully provided many pointers on what officers should look out for amongst their division of sailors. Was anyone particularly camp or effeminate? Was anyone very flamboyant or wearing very stylish or garish clothes? They would certainly merit close attention. Duty officers in HM ships were also required to conduct safety and security patrols or 'Rounds' of the ship, during the middle watch between midnight and 0400, looking for hazards or emergencies in the small hours. Trainee duty officers were taught that a key aspect of these middle watch rounds was to look out for homosexual activity in remote parts of the ship and also for any evidence of such activity. Ingrained in my memory is the very precise description that we were given by training course officers, to look out for broom handles with brown stains. I'll leave it to your imagination as to what these broom handles were supposed to have been used for but needless to say – and thankfully – I never did find one!

When I started writing this chapter I planned on focusing on tales from my warfare officer days, but I've realised that it would be remiss of me not to include an incident that occurred when I was Executive Officer and Second-in-Command of HMS *Lancaster* in the second half of the 1990s. I'd been in post for well over a year, and had taken the ship from the messy depths of refit in Devonport through the stresses of operational sea training and worldwide deployments. This included my first return visit to the Falkland Islands since the conflict in 1982. I'm confident that I played a key role in moulding the ship into a close-knit and cohesive fighting unit with a good reputation in the Fleet. One afternoon, completely out of the blue, I was summoned to the Captain's cabin. The ship

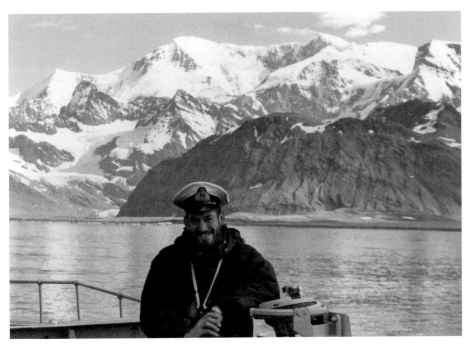

Above: My return to the Falkland Islands in 1996 as XO of HMS *Lancaster*. Fifteen years on, it was amazing to see these islands thriving.

Below: After few port visits and Christmas away from home, we were thrilled to be able to return via Chile and Ecuador and the Panama Canal.

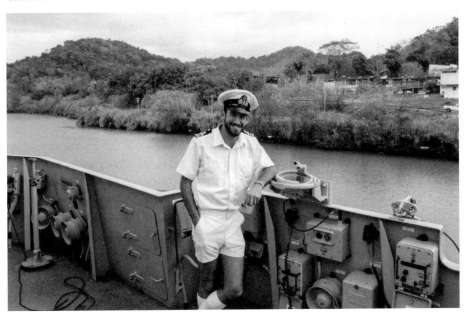

was in UK waters and as I made my way from the ship control centre, where I'd been chatting to the on watch stokers, up three decks to the Captain's personal cabin, I had no idea what he wanted to discuss. The Captain was a delightful man, an easy-going but supremely professional aviator with whom I had an exceptional relationship. We worked very well together – as a command team we had achieved a lot with the ship and we (the ship) had a good reputation in the squadron and the RN more widely. He invited me to sit down and the bombshell then dropped. He'd been approached by an officer on board who had reported that several members of the wardroom were openly discussing whether or not the XO was gay. Apparently I had been observed with a male friend on a number of occasions in different ports and that was enough to spark rumours. Fuck. Dry mouth, heart pounding, sweating profusely – all of the recognisable stress characteristics – descended instantaneously. God knows how but I managed to stay calm and maintain a balanced demeanour, denied the accusation and coolly explained that a pal had been having problems and I'd been helping him deal with some personal issues. The Captain immediately accepted my explanation and we discussed how best to deal with the issue in the wardroom – confront the challenge with a view to putting it to bed or ignore it. My initial response was to ignore it but after thinking about it for a few minutes, I decided to confront the challenge. Having left the CO's cabin, I summoned all officers, including the heads of departments (HoDs), to the wardroom, banished the stewards from the wardroom pantry, closed all the doors to the wardroom and, as calmly as I could, explained what had been reported. Much to my chagrin, I then had to lie to my officers. I denied that I was gay, and said that I was exceptionally disappointed, indeed livid, that such gossip could come from my wardroom, that I had worked fucking hard to get the ship to where it was today and that if the rumours spread around the ship, it would have a significantly negative impact on the ship and be to the detriment of everything that everyone on board had worked so hard for over the last eighteen months. I then left. Actually, I stormed out and declined to eat in the mess that night.

I was intensely angry, both at the potential risk to my career and that everything that I/we had worked so hard together to achieve as a team in the ship could be destroyed. In hindsight, I was also extremely pissed off that I had to turn on myself in order to save face with the team that I worked so well with and also that I was still having to lie about my sexuality at the very end of the twentieth century. I briefed the Captain on my one-way transmission at my wardroom and he commended me on a gutsy call, thus reinforcing my high opinion of him. Fortunately, no more was said and the rumours apparently did not spread around the ship – or if they did, I was unaware. Many years later, I took my CO, by then a retired RN commodore, out to supper. By this time he knew I was gay and we discussed the incident. He was as gracious over supper as he had been at the time – he had had no inkling that I was gay when I was his XO but fully understood why I had denied it at the time.

Fast forward ten or so years. Having had to fight for my career survival in 1996, in 2006 I found myself marching in uniform at the front of Pride London – the first time that UK military had ever marched in uniform in a gay pride parade. Indeed, we think it was the first time that a nation's military had ever marched officially in uniform in a gay pride parade anywhere in the world. Finally I could be myself, an out and very proud serving officer in Her Majesty's Royal Navy, in full view of tens of thousands of people! What an amazing day. The roar that went up from the crowd as we first hove into view on Oxford Street was overwhelming; it sent tingles of exhilaration down my spine and I felt quite choked up. The years of shame and darkness were finally being eclipsed – and in the most spectacular, rainbow-coloured way possible! Everyone had been on tenterhooks about the sort of reception we might get but I can honestly say that, once the crowd realised we weren't all in fancy dress, the response was almost universally and very noisily positive! The small, vocal Christian fundamentalist contingent positioned outside St James's Palace who took umbrage at our presence in uniform didn't stand a chance. They were drowned out by the cheers of the crowd and even more so by the London Fire Brigade fire engine, which was conveniently positioned immediately astern of the military contingent, and which coincidentally (!) sounded their sirens as we passed the small protest group. The effect on the young sailors in the RN platoon was also amazing; several came up to me afterwards to say that for the first time, they felt

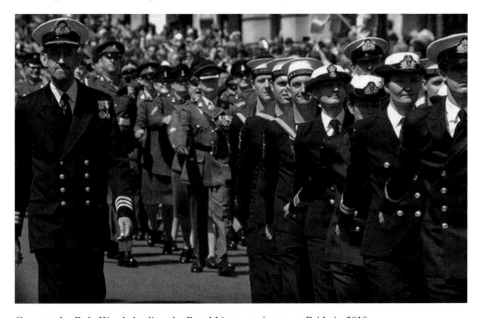

Commander Roly Woods leading the Royal Navy contingent at Pride in 2010.

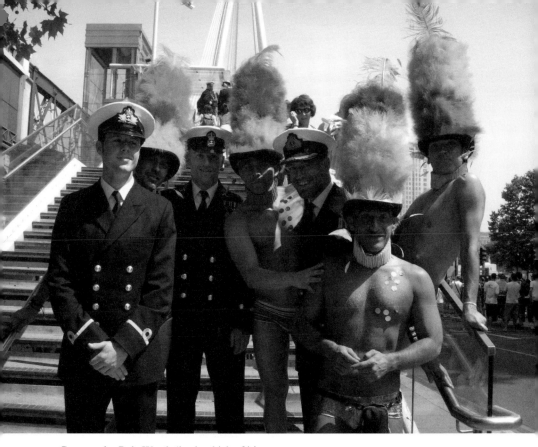

Commander Roly Woods 'in the thick of it'.

fully included and proud to be gay and serving their country – not sentiments that roughy-toughy sailors usually articulate. I won't go into the trials and tribulations of what we went through to be able to participate in Pride London – suffice to say that a massive shout-out is due to Craig Jones, Lady Rosie West, wife of the then First Sea Lord Admiral Alan West, and to Admiral West himself for allowing the RN to literally lead the way. It took another three years before our gay colleagues in the British Army and RAF were authorised to march in uniform at Pride.

In addition to gay pride, we now have a robust RN LGBTQ forum firmly established with CGRM (Commandant General Royal Marines) as the Diversity & Inclusion champion for the RN, D&I reps in every unit and establishment, and we are sufficiently mature as an organisation that posters advertising National Coming Out Day can be confidently displayed without fear of retribution or graffiti.

For all the challenges I had to face during the first half of my career, I've had a blast! I'm still serving in uniform at Navy Ops in Northwood and, as I tell people on a regular basis, having recently celebrated the fortieth anniversary of my arrival at BRNC Dartmouth in September 2018, I can honestly say that I have enjoyed every appointment/assignment immensely. I reckon that if I can say that after four decades of service, then I took the right decision when I jumped on that steam train in 1978.

The Royal Navy taking part in National Coming Out Day, 2018.

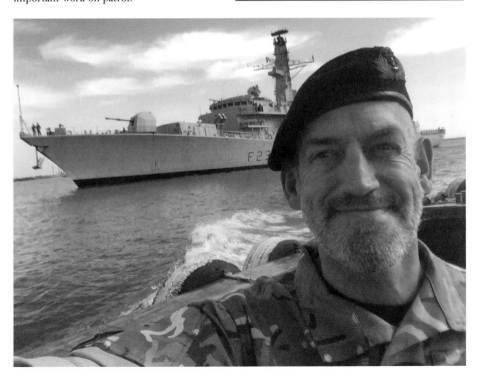

NATIONAL COMING OUT DAY & WORLD MENTAL HEALTH DAY 2018

THE CLOSET IS BAD FOR YOUR HEALTH

Military life is stressful enough, and adding the burden of hiding your sexual orientation or gender identity could be the straw that breaks the camel's back. Work and home life suffer when people in same-sex relationships try to hide their sexual orientation from co-workers.

Morale is improved when sailors and marines can be open and honest about who they are with their oppos - the best dits come from real life!

Don't be the reason your oppo feels forced to stay in the closet - help the Naval Service to create a welcoming and healthy environment for all.

Speak to a doctor or medical assistant if you are experiencing anxiety, depression, or any other mental health issues. Early care is key to a happy life.

NATIONAL COMING OUT DAY — 11 Oct 18

WORLD MENTAL HEALTH DAY — 10 Oct 18

compass the sexual orientation & gender identity network of the Naval Service

Older, wiser and still loving the life at sea. Commander Roly Woods in the Gulf in 2016, helping prepare our ships for their important work on patrol.

Chapter 9

Naivety, Secrecy, Prejudice and Pride
Lieutenant Commander Mandy McBain MBE
Royal Navy

It was with complete excitement that I boarded the train to join the Women's Royal Naval Service in November 1986. This had been an ambition of mine for years, probably ever since joining the Sea Cadets in the late 1970s. In 1986, females couldn't join the WRNS until they were 17½, so knowing that I needed to do something after leaving school at 16, I got a job working at Austin Rover. I never lost sight of my clear ambition to join the WRNS. So, at 19, with my mum and stepdad tearfully waving me off at Coventry station, I started my adventure, and this was how it made me feel: no apprehension, no doubts; just complete excitement. In the bag that had been thrust upon me on my departure, along with far too much food packed by my anxious mother, who clearly thought that

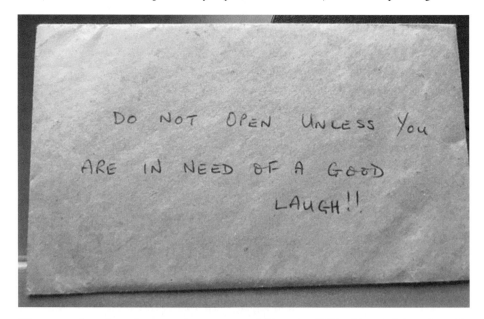

The unopened envelope given to me by my mum on 3 November 1986 as I boarded the train to join the Navy.

rationing was still in place in the military, I found an envelope with a message on the front from my mum saying, 'Do not open unless you are in need of a good laugh'. Clearly this remained intact, as I was living my dream.

I seemed to fit into service life with ease. I loved the rules and regulations and that you knew what you were doing, when you were doing it, and what to wear. Working as a team, doing exercise, assault courses and classroom work, I really was having a ball – and being paid for it! I did think of home but didn't really miss it.

At that time females and males did their training very separately, which always made for an amusing experience when we all met up. I look back now and can see that it was a parade of egos and showmanship with both genders vying for attention. I had left a boyfriend at home who regularly wrote and sent gifts. I returned the kindness occasionally, but, to be honest, I was too busy loving my new life.

From an early stage in my naval career it was obvious that the rules were such that if you were gay you were dismissed from the service. There were always rumours, people talked, had an opinion, and never felt shy in saying how wrong being gay was and how they wouldn't want to serve with anyone like that. I had never met anyone who was gay. I wasn't gay, so it didn't make any difference to me. I remember feeling surprised about the passion with which people condemned being gay.

I didn't really have an opinion about it, but I remember the comedy characters on television that portrayed being gay as different, strange and something to be laughed at.

I remained in Plymouth for my initial and then my specialist training before getting my first 'real' job in Scotland. Now that my primary ambition of joining the WRNS had been achieved and I had completed basic training, having won the Raleigh Medal for being the best recruit in my class, my next goal was beginning to surface. I wanted to be an officer. I didn't have the academic qualifications, but I really felt I was going to achieve it somehow.

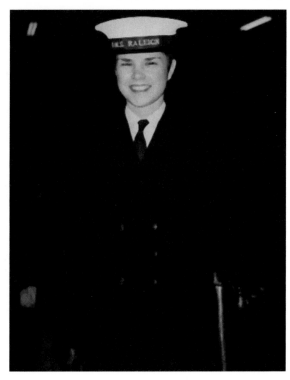

HMS Raleigh, December 1986.

It didn't feel that long ago that I'd left a good job in Civvy Street, which I'd loved, before starting what still seemed like a bit of an adventure. However, now I was at my first non-training naval establishment it did feel different. I remember Faslane Naval Base appearing vast and everyone seemed to know what they were doing – they were confident, appeared to know each other and were all very

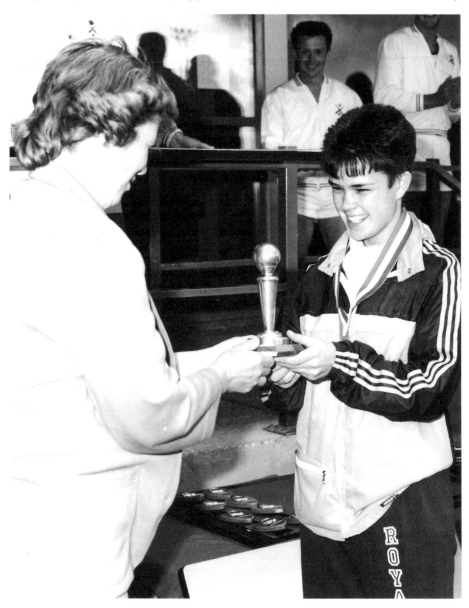

A sports event at Faslane, c.1988.

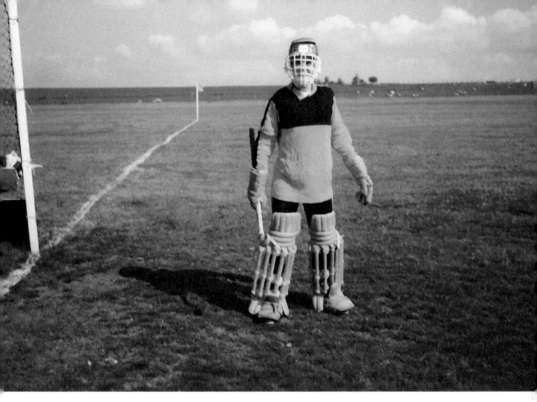

Playing hockey for the establishment, 1988.

funny. I must've looked and sounded every bit like the young newbie. I tried to blend in; I wanted to be liked as I really did feel like a fish out of water. I lived in WRNS quarters and immersed myself in sport, whether it was road running, cross-country, volleyball, athletics, clay pigeon shooting or learning to ski. Most of the time it was a case of 'all the gear, no real idea'!

My life was hectic. I was working to get my professional task book completed, taking private maths lessons to help me gain the missing qualification I needed in order to be considered for selection to attend the Admiralty Interview Board (AIB). The driving force behind all of this was my burning ambition to become an officer in the Women's Royal Naval Service.

As if my life wasn't busy enough, I started seeing a wonderful man who was caring, funny and good-looking, and who thought the world of me. We travelled a fair bit and generally had a great time together. We were a couple for a while, but for me, as much as I cared for him, something didn't make me feel like he was 'the one'. It wasn't fair on him to continue, so I ended it and we parted as friends. As sad as I was with our separation, it gave me time to focus fully on trying to pass my maths exam to enable me to get nearer reaching my ambition.

Maths didn't, and still doesn't, come naturally to me. I became such a regular stressed face in the Education Centre that the lieutenant in charge of the department started to bring me cups of tea to keep me going when I was sitting the exams!

I was well supported by my friends, my seniors and my family back home. They all wanted me to do well and achieve my goal, but all this kindness resulted in extra pressure at times. As well as doing my own maths study, in preparation for becoming an officer I had to attend CW lessons, which stood for commissioning warrant. These were arranged by the establishment and were lessons that *allegedly* prepared you to be an officer. Most of us attended to show willing and because there was a feeling that you had to do them. There was even a rumour that we would be taught how to eat a banana with a knife and fork! Thankfully, that wasn't true.

It was at these lessons that I met another Wren who was also striving to be selected for AIB. We had lots in common, even if much of this was getting comfort from the fact that we both felt like we weren't quite good enough to even be considered for a commission. One of the discussions we had to present to the rest of the group was to report our findings from a newspaper that we had been allocated. I remember it well. Imposter syndrome at the fore, we all sat round a large conference table and I was trying to sound like I knew what I was talking about as I worked my way down the pile of daily papers. I gave a breakdown of the main news from the previous week and then offered my opinion on the headlines, taking convoluted questions from other CW candidates who wanted to impress. However, what I wasn't aware of, working its way to the top of my pile was a porn magazine that had been hidden in there by my ever-supportive friends! I thankfully ended my debrief just one newspaper away from this magazine reaching the top of the pile. This would have been a lesson not to forget and a sure-fire way of not being selected to go any further.

In between all this coaching/classroom work, I was immersing myself fully into establishment life, helping out and volunteering for events. It was decided that there would be a Christmas disco in the WRNS block. I offered to be the main organiser but roped in a few other people to help me. It was for charity and we made it fancy dress, charging people for the privilege of attending. The event was packed; all ranks and rates attended, and we raised a lot of money, but it was hard work with all the organising, lifting and shifting. I ended up hurting my back, but it was the offer of a healing massage from a fellow Wren that changed my life forever.

I was in shock; I'd never really thought of myself as being gay, but I was completely enjoying the attention of another woman. And for both of us, it was our first same-sex relationship. We knew from the very start we had to keep it completely secret. Nobody at all knew. Like every new relationship, it was exciting, but on the other hand, completely terrifying as we were under no illusions about the consequences of being found out. There was always talk about who people thought might be gay. We heard of raids and people being drafted to other establishments at short notice or being investigated, interviewed and detained for days on end. I really don't know if any of this was true, but it was certainly a way of making us keep our relationship absolutely secret. We quickly learnt to skilfully balance living in two separate worlds, creating a persona that people saw and believed. This was helped by us being adept at speaking in the third person, learning to avoid direct questions about what we did in our spare time and living lives of make-believe and, on many occasions, lying. It was balanced with our own time when we were together and free from prying eyes, ears and the Special Investigation Branch (SIB). The hardest part was lying to those whom we respected and who respected us.

At times it was exhausting trying to remember what we did, who we had told. With all of this in the background, I was still trying to gain my maths qualification. After three attempts at the exam, I finally passed, but the annoying thing was that the exam markers staged a strike, so I didn't get the results of the first exam before I had to register and take the next one. In the end, I actually passed it twice! Within weeks of this momentous result I was in Portsmouth attending my Admiralty Interview Board.

Although nervous, I was full of excitement again as I'd finally made it, after what seemed like an age since joining the WRNS three years earlier. In preparation for the AIB, I remember having to buy a suit as I didn't own one. However, before doing this I had to apply for a credit card to enable me to get it. The whole AIB experience was a challenge, that's for sure, not to mention that, after all the faff of getting a new suit, there was another candidate wearing exactly the same one. And to top it all, we were on the same small selection panel so followed each other round for the two days like twins.

The final interview was something that I had heard so much about – mainly horror stories. But for me, the interview with the WRNS officer, who was the Personnel Selection Officer, was the one I dreaded the most. This was a less formal interview, more of a one-to-one chat. They asked about drugs, finances … and the dreaded gay question. They also wanted to make sure you were under no illusions about what the rules were in the Navy at that time. I managed to get through this interview and the rest of my AIB and was successful. I was overjoyed, excited and nervous at the thought of what may lie ahead. I was selected to join Britannia Royal Naval College, Dartmouth (BRNC) in the November, which was only a few months away.

At that time, WRNS officer candidates only did three months at Dartmouth; because females didn't go to sea, the training was shorter. I can't say BRNC was particularly enjoyable, but I got through it, using my 'days to go' chart on the back of my wardrobe door to keep me going. The whole experience felt like more of what I imagined a finishing school to be like rather than a military college. Many of the activities were tailored to be an inconvenience to try to make them comparable to what our male colleagues had to go through. For example, when we

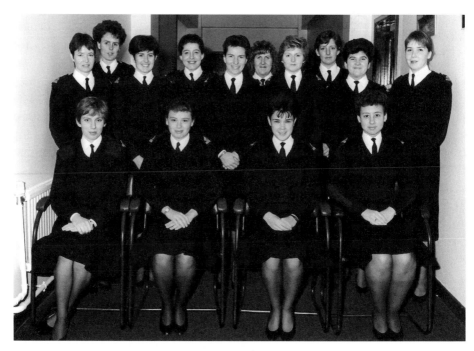

BRNC Dartmouth, Talbot Division Class, December 1989.

A press release from BRNC Dartmouth to announce my award of the Pauline Doyle Trophy for 'Prowess on the Parade Ground whilst retaining one's femininity', 1989.

61.

Britannia Royal Naval College
PRESS RELEASE

Prowess on the Parade Ground whilst retaining one's femininity is the quality required to win the Pauline Doyle Trophy.

A former pupil of Stoke Lodge School at Coventry, Mandy McBain (22) has passed out from the Britannia Royal Naval College this month (16 December) as a WRNS Officer and took the Trophy in her stride.

Her parents Sheila and John Eaton live in Keresley and travelled down to Dartmouth to watch the Commandant General Royal Marines take the Salute at the Passing Out Parade when one hundred and twenty seven young Officers successfully completed their College course.   Mrs Min Kingston, Mandy's Grandmother also made the long journey to offer her congratulations.

During her three months at Dartmouth Mandy joined over four hundred male counterparts. Her academic and professional course comprised Naval History, Current Affairs, Supply and Management, boat handling on the River Dart and Parade Training as well as learning about the Women's Royal Naval Service.

were on Dartmoor for two days, carrying what felt like our own body weight in a rucksack while being assessed on leadership tasks and trekking for miles, each morning all of the females were inspected to make sure we were wearing make-up. On our kit list was combat green eyeshadow, which we were expected to wear. The staff justified this by saying that male students had to shave, so therefore we were to wear make-up. This was an extra trauma for me as I didn't actually own any make-up at that time, let alone combat green eyeshadow!

During my time at BRNC, my secret relationship continued, but it was a matter of balancing the socially acceptable image of being seen with a man at the right time in the right place, attending functions and talking about boyfriends, alongside following my feelings that were so far removed from this image that I had to create. It was tiring and took a lot of planning.

Just before I graduated from BRNC, the government announced that for the first time, females would start serving at sea. This was not driven by the Admiralty wanting equality for females; it was as a result of the falling numbers in recruitment of men, which meant that ships were undermanned. Going to sea was something that, to be honest, I had never even thought I would have the chance to do. Whilst I didn't have to make a decision about my future immediately, as I'd not completed officer training, I knew it was a choice that I would have to make before too long.

My first job as a WRNS officer was back in Scotland as a correspondence officer for a submarine in refit. My secret relationship continued, but I did feel lucky as my girlfriend was also now based in Scotland. We continued to live a very complex life of travelling and editing, and seeing each other when we could and spending most leave periods together. It was also during this time that all serving females were asked to make a decision about going to sea. Because I joined up prior to this ruling, I had reserved rights, which meant I was given the choice about going to sea. I made the decision not to volunteer. However, I know that if this opportunity had been offered to me a few years earlier, I would have jumped at the chance. But now I was in a same-sex relationship in a service that would dismiss me if I was to be found out. I surmised that going to sea would only highlight my difference; living cheek to cheek with many other people 24/7 would make it all the more difficult to blend in, to hide the fact that I was in a relationship with another woman. The atmosphere at the time felt toxic: the voices of the serving men who didn't want us to work alongside them at sea were clear. The leadership from the top was not convincing and a few years later, I saw an internal memorandum written by the then Second Sea Lord (Head of HR) that stated: 'the changes would have the benefit of improving the scope for the equality of opportunity and contribution' for women. However, he then went on to warn that 'There are also counterarguments: culture shock, spouses' resistance, emotional tensions developing within crews, weakening of the male self-image …

and unpredictability of women's availability because of pregnancy.' The lack of convincing leadership and positive messages alongside my own concerns of being found out and dismissed made the decision an easy one. I didn't want to put any more pressure on myself so the decision to become a 'non-sea volunteer' was made and would be with me for the rest of my career.

During my appointment in Scotland, my stepfather was taken ill and after a short illness, he passed away. It was an incredible blow to me, but more so because I was, and still am, so very close to my mum and I felt I knew how much she would be hurting, especially after the death of my father about ten years beforehand. It brought us much closer together. I still hadn't told her about my relationship, but right now certainly didn't feel like the appropriate time. I didn't like the thought of my mum being on her own and I enjoyed her company, so many leave periods were spent with both my mum and my girlfriend. They got on very well, but surprisingly, Mum never asked anything about our relationship. After a few more years, I decided it was time to come out to my mum. The task before me felt huge as I was risking losing the love and respect of not just my mum, but my role model, my coach and mentor, and my best friend. I packed

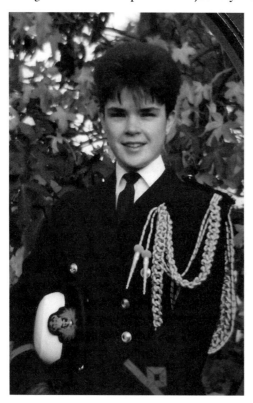

a bag in case she asked me to leave and told her that my girlfriend was more than a friend. Mum hadn't picked up on any of this, which I still find hard to believe as she is a very astute woman. She was completely unfazed, and when I told her I had a bag packed, she asked me where I was going. I don't remember much more about this event, apart from it all being OK, but I knew that I was lucky as I had heard of one awful coming-out story where a family had disowned their daughter. As stressful as this situation was, my 'Do not open unless you are in need of a good laugh' envelope remained intact.

My career took some unpredictable turns and I was called for an interview with the Commander-in-Chief-Fleet to see if I would be suitable to work in his outer office. I was selected and this

As Third Officer and PA to the Commander-in-Chief Fleet (CINCFLEET), 1991.

therefore meant moving from Scotland to Northwood, near London, to be a

PA to a four-star admiral. I loved this job. It was hard work with long hours, but by this time, my girlfriend had also moved out of Scotland, so at least the commute to see each other when we could was slightly easier. The double life continued to be exhausting: conversations, periods of leave and weekends that were allegedly spent with other friends, family or fictitious boyfriends at home – all these people rarely had a service connection to avoid any cross-checking.

I eventually moved to the south coast for my next job. This time, my girlfriend was appointed many miles away, which made travelling to see each other more difficult. Along with leading a double life, we both had elements of weekend working, new interests, new friends and our own careers to balance. All of this took its toll, and after many years of hiding our relationship, it came to an end. It was so hard hiding the hurt and sadness of finishing a relationship. I felt so alone, as I didn't have anyone to talk to. Work had to continue, as did my sporting commitments and everything else. I had to appear to be totally unfazed. It was now that I felt I needed to come out to a few very close friends. It was normally on a night out, after a few drinks, that I would feel brave enough to reveal some, not all, details, but mainly, the headliner that I was gay. This didn't faze the few I told, and I am fairly sure they had suspected something, but for them it didn't matter. I was aware that I had burdened them with my secret, as at that time they could have also been asked about me by the Special Investigation Branch (SIB).

During my time in this job I received a letter to say that I had been selected for a vetting interview. I remember the sinking feeling and being consumed with worry about it. A big part of the vetting process is an interview that you must pass in order to be able to see things, hear things and work on documents that are classified Secret and above. Not everyone is vetted, but in my current role I was likely to have access to such documents. The vetting interview is an experience that most people dread as it is so intrusive. It consists of a one-to-one exchange, supposedly more informal to encourage you to open up about things you probably wouldn't even tell your best friend. A written record is taken at the time and it is this report that can mean the difference between you being successfully granted a higher security clearance or not. During the awkward chat with the total stranger, you are asked to reveal everything about your finances, your friends, your personal relationships, your sex life, where you have travelled to, why and with whom, while they look at your passport. With the rules as they were at that time, my sexuality was not something that I was about to reveal to a stranger, especially considering most of my close friends didn't even know, and to do so would end my career.

I was terrified at the thought of this ordeal. I might have become an expert at talking in the third party, avoiding questions almost daily, but in a one-to-one interview, sat across the desk from someone who does this every day, it was not going to be as easy.

As an added bonus, I needed to hide the fact that I had recently returned from flying to Malta to meet my then girlfriend over the New Year period – a risky business at the best of times, but just unlucky this close to my interview. It wouldn't have taken much to look at what ships were alongside and where to notice that this may have been more than a coincidence. I had primed my wonderfully loyal mum to be on standby in case they asked her if we had spent the New Year on holiday together. Thankfully, she wasn't needed. For this process I had to nominate referees who would be interviewed about me. Whilst my sexuality was something that I had never discussed with my friend Cherry, I always knew that she had an idea. She is a very organised person and therefore wanted to make sure she knew everything she was supposed to know prior to her interview, so we talked in riddles about which man I was seeing, what he looked like and when we had last been out etc. Cherry was based at another establishment and was being interviewed immediately prior to my own.

I had been so aware of the time and what she would have been going through, and I was astonished to hear from her as soon as her interview was over and the Vetting Officer had just left her office. Her first words were, 'How tall are you?' She repeated that question until I answered '5'3''. She then burst out laughing as she had told the VO that I was 5'9"! She had admitted to not knowing the colour of my eyes or what my father's occupation was, apart from dead – her words, not mine! He probably left feeling confused as to whether they were even talking about the same person, let alone discussing my possible sexuality. I received my Developed Vetting and ironically never got to view anything above a Secret classification at all!

All of this editing, thinking and overthinking situations just became part of my everyday life, so much so that I probably didn't even notice I was doing it half of the time. I was still enjoying my life and started playing volleyball for the Navy. This brought with it a completely new circle of friends, including many civilians whom I would not otherwise have met. It was through this circle that I became aware of the father of one of my civilian friends who was a warrant officer in the Navy and had been seconded to the HPAT, which was the Homosexuality Policy Assessment Team. In 1996, they were tasked with undertaking a review of the military policy and the anticipated effects on fighting power if homosexuals were integrated into the Armed Forces. Rumour of this team and what they were trying to achieve was rife; people were worried but had no way of asking about it without fearing that their interest would make their sexuality obvious.

I was approached by my friend, on behalf of her father, to see if I would consider being interviewed by him for the report. I remember feeling this was something I needed to do, especially as it turned out that most of the other report writers didn't have access to any serving lesbian, gay or bisexual people, therefore our voices would never be heard or taken into consideration in the report. I agreed to do this but only at a neutral place, and obviously that my identity would not be revealed. I think it helped him understand the fact that we wanted to be offered the same opportunities as our heterosexual colleagues without fearing that we would be dismissed from a service that I strangely still felt loyal towards. I never saw his version of our interview.

After months of speculation, the report was published and asserted that to allow gays in the military would be bad for morale and leave them vulnerable to blackmail from foreign intelligence agencies. I remember the bitter disappointment that I felt at this result. It really did feel like it was one step forwards and many steps backwards if they were still using the 'vulnerable to blackmail' statement. I felt that having to hide so much about myself made me more prone to being blackmailed. I had gone from feeling empowered to be able to contribute in some way to the report to feeling helpless, hopeless and isolated again.

About every two years I was reappointed, and this time was given a job that pushed me out of my comfort zone, but in the end, I loved. It was at the Admiralty Interview Board and I was one of three personnel selection officers. It was strange going back there and rather ironic being the person who would conduct the more personal interview, which included a chat to make sure the candidates were aware of the military's stance on not allowing LGB people into the services and the consequences if they were. I never had anyone telling me they were gay, but my question set was probably very short!

I had started to see a civilian girl and it was extremely hard at times to get her to comprehend how serious our situation was for me and what the penalties would be if we were found out. She just couldn't really understand the need to talk in the third party and keep everything so discreet and secret when we were in company. One thing I know for sure: it was an added strain on our relationship. I worked for a commodore who was an inspiration, a real gent and a delight to work for. We got on well and had a lot of mutual respect for each other. We were in the section that dealt with the cases when people had been found out to be either lesbian or gay and raised the paperwork to dismiss them accordingly. I don't mention bisexual as I don't recall ever seeing a case of anyone being dismissed for being bi.

I remember a young woman asking to have a meeting with me, and it turned out that the department I was in had previously raised the paperwork for her dismissal. She wanted to lodge a complaint against being dismissed from the Navy in case the rules changed in the future and she wanted to rejoin. I can remember being quite shocked and wondering why she had chosen me to help her write it, but I was never brave enough to ask that question. I helped her write her letter, but I don't know what happened or whether she asked to rejoin once the rules changed.

My job was interesting, and the Commodore was very keen for me to learn as much as possible. I remember one day when I was not allowed into some of his meetings, which was unusual. The closed-door sessions all looked serious and the atmosphere felt restrained, especially when a naval barrister was called to his office. Towards the end of the day, I was asked to come into the boss's office for an interview. His 2IC was with him and I was asked if I wanted to have anyone with me at this meeting. It was all a bit strange as I didn't know, for sure, what it was about, although I did have that dreaded feeling that this could be the one interview I had been avoiding for the majority of my career.

I declined the offer to have anyone with me. My heart was racing; I felt sick. My boss explained that it had been reported to the department that I was in a relationship with a female. He wanted reassurance that I knew what the consequences were if this was true. He asked me whether I was seeing a female who was also in the Navy. I answered, correctly, no. As soon as I heard this question I knew his intelligence was incorrect as I was actually seeing a female civilian. This gave me an inner strength, although I was shaking to the core.

I really can't recall how long I was in there for, but it did feel like an awful long time. My boss ended the interview once I had assured him I was not in a lesbian relationship with another serving female. He then told me to go home and pour myself a big gin and tonic. This whole situation couldn't have been pleasant for him, either; it was one of those awful loops that he had to do something about and I had to endure. I think my respect for him increased after this ordeal, as strange as that might sound. I felt he conducted the whole interview in a very diplomatic and respectful way. I knew I had been lucky.

As in the normal appointing cycle, I moved on to another job, again in the Portsmouth Naval Base. The legal battle to get the rules changed for LGB people in the UK military was continuing in the background. It was often covered on the TV news, and whilst I wanted to look interested, it very much depended on where I was or who I was with as to how engaged I appeared. Everyone was becoming more aware that it was highly likely that there would be changes to the current rules, but no one knew what they would be like. The department I worked in at that time was tasked with contacting every ship to find out what the feelings were if LGB people were allowed to serve in the future. My job was to collate all of the returns and summarise them into a report. Some of the comments were just ridiculous, so much so that I edited to my complete satisfaction. As an example, I remember reading one comment from a commanding officer who was concerned that 'they' would want to dance together at functions and what action should be taken if 'they' kissed. Another concern was that the ship would have to pay for an additional gay TV channel. It was like reading comments from people who had never met anyone who was gay and that gay people were so different to them that they would behave in an unacceptable and embarrassing way.

At this time, I was working for what can only be described as a homophobic and misogynistic senior officer. One day he commented on the fact that he felt I didn't seem to be at all concerned by the possibility of the rules changing. Well, I wasn't, especially in comparison to how horrified he was at the thought of serving beside openly LGB people. He went on to describe what he thought would be an awful situation for me to experience, in a bid to get me to understand how dreadful the change would be for me and others in the future. He asked me to 'imagine how you would feel having to live and sleep in a mess deck with a lot of lesbians'.

If only he knew!

At this point, being a non-sea volunteer, I nearly changed my mind.

It wasn't long after this comment that the European Court of Human Rights overruled the military. I can remember exactly where I was when I heard the announcement on the radio that people currently serving would no longer be dismissed from the military for being gay. Lesbians and bisexuals didn't really get much of a mention, but the news was absolutely amazing, all the same. Although there had been lots of speculation that this would be the case, it still felt like a huge weight had been lifted off my shoulders. Whilst I really wasn't ready to come out to the world, it did mean that I didn't have to worry about losing the job I loved and my pension, or having to go through a dreadful investigation by SIB. I'm not quite sure what people expected would happen after the announcement, but there was a lot of talk about this decision at the time. Even so, the language I was hearing still sounded homophobic; it certainly didn't make me want to reveal anything. I also had the personal battle to wrestle with as I had lied for many years to the people I worked with, my friends and my family. How would they take it if I came out to them and said that, actually, the persona I had carried off was not me at all? It was an act that they may not understand was necessary, having to weigh up whether people would engage with me or dismiss and disown me. I remember, a few years later, somebody saying that when you come out, that is the point when you're actually ready to take the risk that, from this time onwards, you may lose that particular friendship or relationship forever.

I don't recall many people coming out after the ruling but, over time, I became more aware of other LGB people in the military. It was wonderful having the choice between secrecy and privacy over whether I told people about my sexual orientation. I became aware of a website called Proud2Serve, which was like an underground way of serving LGB people communicating safely with each other. I did look at it but didn't use it very much. I was still very private. Nothing really changed for me until about 2004, when I became aware that there was going to be a meeting of serving LGBT people and this was bizarrely going to be held at the Armed Forces Chaplaincy Centre in Amport. I put my name down not really knowing what this was all about. It was held over a weekend to make it easy for those attendees who perhaps were not out to be there without having to ask for time away from their primary role. It all felt very clandestine. There were about thirty-five of us at the meeting and some of us had our partners there, whether they were serving or not. I still couldn't help feeling slightly suspicious as the HR Policy Officer was also in attendance for the whole weekend. Lieutenant Commander Craig Jones was the motivation behind this initial meeting but also afterwards when taking things forward, such as seeking permission for the Navy to march in uniform at Pride London the following year. The Navy was the first of all three services to be allowed to march in uniform; the other two services had to wear branded T-shirts. During the conference I bravely put my hand up to say I would attend Pride, probably convinced that it would never happen. But it did, and I feel slightly ashamed to say that I didn't feel brave enough to attend. On the day, I sought out every bit of news coverage I could find and a bit of me wished I'd had the confidence to go.

The LGBT meetings continued on a yearly basis and at the next meeting I was asked by the same policy officer to come away with actions, one of which was to form an LGBT network. I can remember sitting there with about six other individuals talking about how we were going to take this forward. With the Navy being a hierarchical organisation, it was felt that it should be somebody with some influence leading it. Looking at the blank faces that were looking back at me, it seemed to be a given that as the only officer there, it was going to be me!

For various reasons, I still didn't attend Pride London until 2008. This was the year that all three services were going to be allowed to march in uniform together for the first time. It was going to be quite historic, so I put my name down to attend. Because it was such a momentous occasion, Pride London put all three services at the very front of the parade. As the Navy is the most senior of

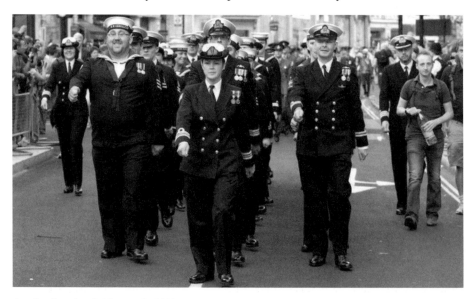

Another London Pride march, 2011.

the three services, we were in front of the Army and RAF. I was the most senior naval person attending and therefore I was also made the parade commander for the Navy.

There could not have been a more public outing than my first-ever Pride London with me being at the front of the whole parade, only preceded by Boris Johnson and other people classed as VIPs. During the parade, the military take a slight diversion towards the end of the march and file past the Cenotaph to pay their respects. We had to wait until the road was cleared by the police. We stopped and waited. I took this opportunity to speak to the naval contingent and remind them that what we had just taken part in was the fun bit, but this next part was for all of those who could never have imagined having this opportunity. A young sailor asked me what I meant by that comment, and it was at this point I realised that we needed to make sure people didn't forget the struggles of those who had gone before us. Many assumed that, as we had marched at Pride, LGBT people being included in the military was a done deal.

What I was now discovering was that the more visible I and the LGBT forum became, the more people contacted me. The network was growing. However, so were some incidences of people being bullied and still not feeling that they had access to the same rights as their heterosexual colleagues. The military didn't recognise partnerships unless you were married, i.e. in a legal partnership. This meant that you didn't have access to married quarters, compassionate leave or, in some cases, the right to bring your partner to social events. Even when civil partnerships came into effect, the rules and regulations took time to be updated. The LGBT forum was now becoming an essential conduit for information to and from the Policy Desk. As the chairperson, I was often consulted on changes and how things should be taken forward. It was empowering to work with those in the LGBT network who were happy to have their voices and opinions heard.

The Navy was the first of the three services to join Stonewall's Diversity Champions programme in 2005. This offered a way for the Navy to get advice on best LGB practice and to be able to network with other organisations. I was allowed to attend Stonewall's Workplace Conferences, which I did for many years as the Navy's only representative. Looking around me, it became apparent that others from the Navy Policy Team should also be attending. Whilst I was in a position of some influence, it was limited. My attendance, especially when I was in uniform, generated much interest, and I was asked to talk to many different organisations about the progress on LGBT inclusion that had been made by the Navy since the military's standing start in 2000. My first-ever public speaking event was at The Law Society Hall, a daunting place in itself. I remember feeling sick with nerves as the audience of about 200 filed in, but everything I said went down very well and I was asked many questions. I loved the whole experience, as well as the attention afterwards, which, I must admit, was completely unexpected.

There seemed to be a real thirst to hear about my story and learn about the progress that was ongoing in the Navy. There was also disbelief that people were being investigated and dismissed up until 2000, with many thinking I was referring to pre-Second World War days. From then I thought I could and would make a difference. Feedback from these types of external engagements presented to my seniors and the Policy Team started to make them much more interested in what I was saying and doing, and the impact that this could be having on the service. Thankfully, I had undergone media training, so this did help my case when justifying my activities, and confirmed that I could be trusted to be a voice for the Navy. The response resulted in the senior officers gradually becoming more engaged and I was increasingly called upon to brief them personally if they were going to attend or speak at conferences. I remember having a conversation with a commodore who said, 'I don't really care what you do in the bedroom,' at which point we had quite a frank conversation about me not caring what he did in the bedroom, either, and pointing out that he had the luxury of not having to hide his relationship and could choose to be private without being forced into secrecy.

Gradually there was more senior attendance at the Stonewall conference through better understanding of why the military must look more inclusive to attract and retain talent. This penny didn't drop quickly, though, which, at times, I found frustrating, but in 2009, I was privileged to be tasked to write the speech for the Second Sea Lord when he was one of the key speakers at the Stonewall Workplace Conference. I remember sitting in the audience feeling so incredibly proud that things had moved so far, and that only nine years after the ban was lifted, one of the most senior leaders in charge of all personnel in the Navy was talking at an LGB conference. I was also very pleased that hardly anything that I had written had been changed; perhaps I was being recognised as a subject matter expert, at last. The senior engagement has continued to increase over subsequent years.

Just after this conference, I left the UK as I was appointed to be the European Forces spokesperson in Sarajevo, Bosnia for six months. An overseas job was not something I had considered in the past, but this came just at the right time as my civil partnership had failed and I had no immediate ties back home. I felt I needed time to find myself again, so I put on hold making the decision not to come back for the full six months. I did have friends fly out to see me, as the country was much safer than it had previously been. I absolutely relished the job and the experiences it gave me. While I was out of the UK, I was still receiving emails as the chairperson of the LGBT forum, and even from that distance, I was able to carry out various engagements. I did an interview with and an article for *The Independent* and I was approached by an editor working with the US Department of Defense to contribute to a book called *Managing Diversity in the Military: the value of inclusion in a culture of uniformity*, and this was published just after my return.

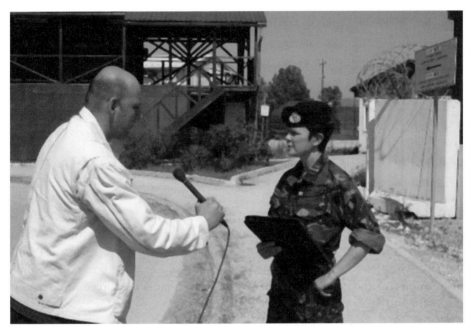

Above: Giving a press interview as the European Forces spokesperson outside Camp Butmir, Sarajevo, following an operation to find Radovan Karadžić, May 2009.

Below: Me with my interpreter during Persons Indicted for War Crimes (PIFWC) operations, May 2009.

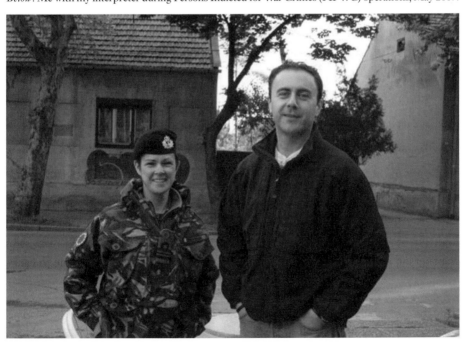

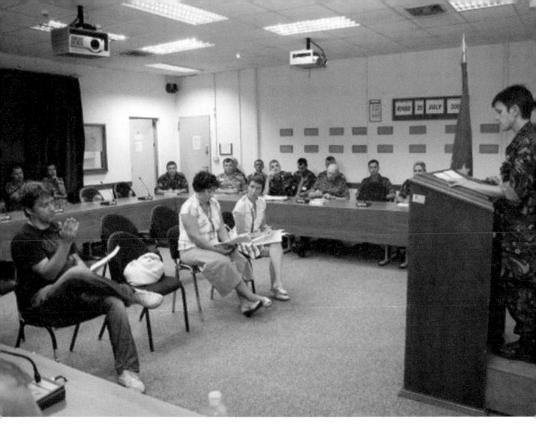

Above: Giving a media briefing (while standing on a box!) in Camp Butmir, Sarajevo, June 2009.

Below: Visiting Bihac, Bosnia, June 2009.

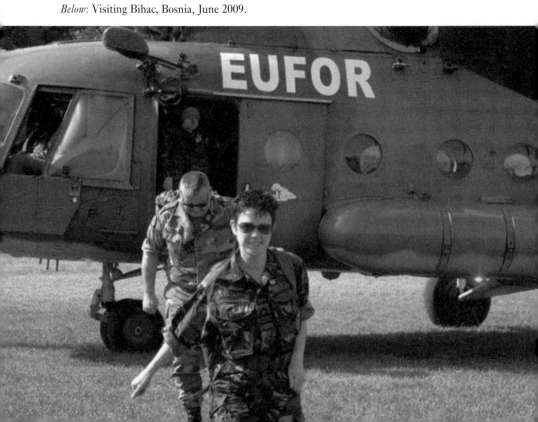

Previously, the Navy had been contacted by an LGBT group in the Netherlands who wanted to start a NATO LGBT forum. A conference was organised and I was selected to attend as the UK military and MoD representative. It was an amazing opportunity to be given the chance to speak at a conference in The Hague. This annual opportunity arose again while I was in Bosnia, and the Navy arranged for me to be flown to Amsterdam to attend. However, this time I had to be quite careful about whom I told back in Sarajevo as there were still some other nations that I was working quite closely with who did not allow LGBT people to serve openly.

During my time in Sarajevo, I experienced personally for the first time an example of homophobic bullying. It completely threw me, probably more so because the very sad thing was that it was by a more senior UK military officer. This person had been using inappropriate words to describe weak situations and people. So, whilst it wasn't directed at me, the colleagues I was working with, who knew I was gay, felt as uncomfortable as I did. Unfortunately, none of them took any action to address this, so I felt I had to. I left the UK as an open, confident and out individual, but at the time I knocked on the door of this senior officer, I was shaking. It was a very stark reminder of how people without rank on their

On the military barge during Amsterdam Pride, 2011.

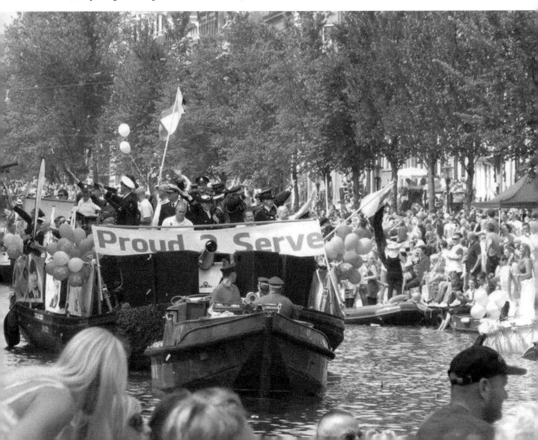

shoulders must feel in a situation like this. It wasn't made any easier when his initial response was that he had been in the military for over thirty years and I was not likely to change him overnight! We discussed it further, I made my point, and he never used homophobic language in front of me again.

On my return from Bosnia, my job was in the policy team in the Royal Navy HQ working on the Equality and Diversity desk. Amongst other things, my portfolio included LGBT inclusion. This meant that I had the pleasure of attending the conference again, but this time it was wearing my LGBT forum and E&D Policy Officer hats. It was 2011, and the Dutch military were being allowed to join Amsterdam's annual Pride parade for the first time, wearing their uniform and having their own boat. I was one of two non-Dutch attendees and, along with Lieutenant Dan Choi from the US Army, had the privilege of cutting a pink feather boa to start the procession of boats. It was a real 'pinch me' moment. The whole experience was incredible and the parade was watched by hundreds of thousands

Being interviewed by the Dutch media with Lieutenant Dan Choi USN before starting Amsterdam Pride, 2011.

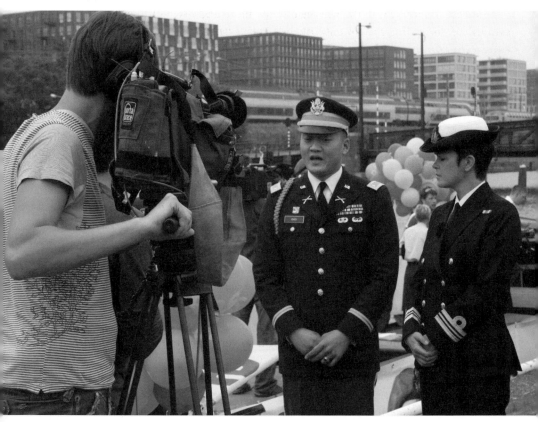

of spectators. On the boat were Dutch generals and other senior officers; some were gay and others were just showing their solidarity. It still seems strange to me that LGBT people had served openly in Dutch units since 1974, but this was the first time that they were allowed to do this in uniform. I gave several interviews on TV, and our presence was covered positively and extensively in the written press. Sometimes I would reflect on the changes I'd seen throughout my career and how I was now being employed to work on LGBT inclusion. It was quite ironic to think that I was on the desk that used to prepare the files to dismiss LGB people.

The following year would be my twenty-fifth in the Royal Navy. As much as I still enjoyed being in the service, I was getting tired of the worry of where my next job might be and whether I would have to move home again. I owned a house on the south coast and really did quite enjoy living in it. And being a non-sea volunteer, this limited the roles I was offered. The chance of redundancy was available, so after much consideration, I decided to apply. I was lucky enough to be selected and started my preparations to leave. Just before Christmas leave in 2011, I was called in by one of my seniors and given an envelope, but was told not to open it until I got home so that I could share the contents with my nearest and dearest. I opened it in the presence of my mum and my then girlfriend. I was astonished on reading the contents of the letter: I had been given an MBE! It was so hard to take this in, to believe what I was reading, especially as I didn't really know why. The text of the letter described me as a widely acclaimed champion of the LGBT community who was unafraid to stand up and be counted. It seemed so ironic to be reading in black and white the words that, for so many years, I had been too afraid to say in full or out loud.

The letter went on to say that I had improved the quality of the workplace and social fabric of the Naval Service and had directly influenced operational capability (OC). The irony in this statement was so hard to digest. For many years, we gays, lesbians and bi serving people had been told that our 'lifestyles' were completely incompatible with the Naval Service and would undermine OC!

For so many years I had lived that exhausting life of make-believe and having to lie to those whom I respected and who respected me in order to remain in the service.

So I left the Navy after twenty-five years' service in March 2012, and the last time I wore my uniform was to receive my MBE, which felt like a very fitting closure to my naval career. Even on the day there was an expectation in the back of my mind that they might decide they had made a mistake! I felt very emotional on the morning of my investiture. It was still so very hard to take it in that I had been nominated for my diversity work, my wanting full inclusion of all of those people that the Navy had hunted down, interrogated, terrified and isolated. During the morning there was a lot of waiting around, which gave me time to reflect on how lucky I had been. I was accompanied by my mum, my partner and

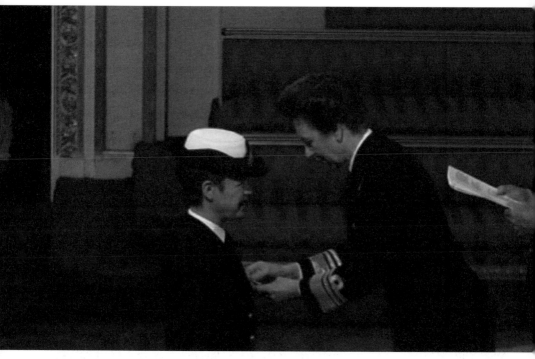

My investiture at Buckingham Palace, May 2012.

one of my best friends. We arrived very early at Buckingham Palace to enable us to appreciate the whole experience as much as possible. However, it was quite strange that while chatting to other recipients of awards, I found myself again being quite reticent about the reason I was receiving mine. This was either, perhaps, through unconscious modesty or, more realistically, my way of protecting myself from a possible shun or having to explain why this was still necessary. Thinking back to how I found myself dumbing down the truth of why I was there, it is amazing how you act after years of avoidance.

I was presented my MBE by the Princess Royal, who is the Chief Commandant for women in the Royal Navy. As a service person, only your rank and name is read out when you are called up to be addressed, so the audience don't know why you are receiving the honour. The Princess Royal asked me why I was there, and I told her it was for the work that I had taken forward in the Navy for full inclusion of lesbian, gay, bi and trans serving people. She replied that sometimes it makes things worse when you highlight differences. We did have a discussion but there was a firm time limit on the chat!

I started working for Stonewall immediately on leaving the Navy but adjusting to life as a civvy was interesting. It wasn't a matter of if I should come out at work; it was more a matter of what I should wear to the office! After twenty-five years of being in uniform, I found it hard to adjust to having the freedom to wear colour.

I joined the membership team as a client account manager but knew I didn't want to work in London, so I became one of the first Stonewall employees to operate remotely. I was given the Defence and Security Sector to manage but also the Diversity Champion organisations based on the south coast. I work with the British Army, Royal Navy, Royal Air Force, Ministry of Defence and other defence-based organisations. My continued work with the military offers me the

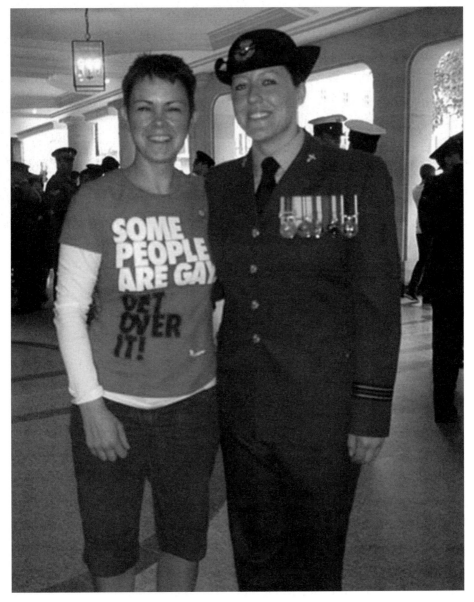

In my civilian job at Stonewall, with Sherry at London Pride, 2014.

chance to work with them, sharing best practice and ensuring that they continue to move forward, which they are achieving at a greater pace each year.

It was through a combination of my previous military links and my continued engagement with the services that I met my now wife, Sherry. We had known each other for many years but our paths never properly crossed until Stonewall needed someone to speak at the annual Workplace Conference. Someone had dropped out at short notice so I was asked to contact Squadron Leader Sherry Conway, who had previously been on a Stonewall Leadership Programme so was considered to be a trusted alumni. Without the added pressures of us being in different services, we really did click. I realised that Sherry was as passionate about LGBT equality as I was and after several meetings, we started dating. Sherry was deployed to Afghanistan three months after we got together. The separation was a challenge, but it was made so much easier because we didn't have to hide our relationship as had been the case for both of us over previous years. We got married in 2016; it was not a small affair, by any means. We had a nearly all-female military guard

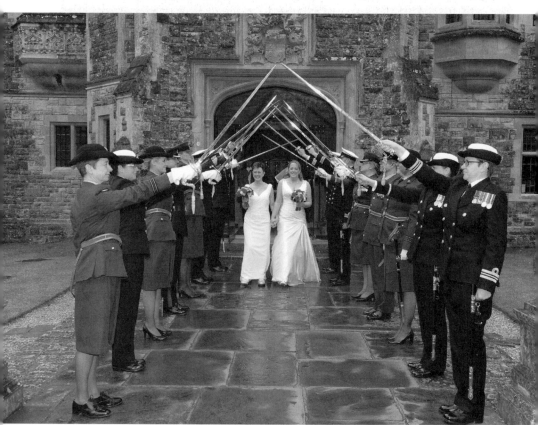

With Sherry on our wedding day, 24 March 2016, in the New Forest.

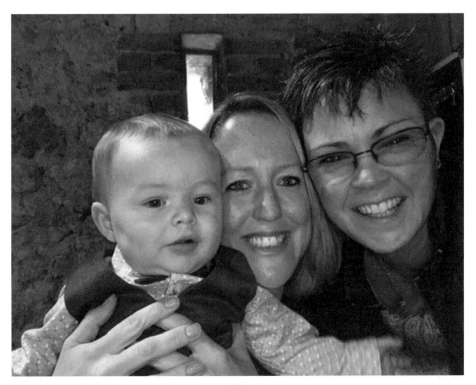

Me, Sherry and Harrison, September 2018.

of honour from the three services. Our wedding was covered by the local press and is featured in a book about women in the Royal Navy. We now have our son, Harrison, who was born in 2018. Sherry is still serving in the RAF and has just returned to work after maternity leave. All of these events and our future together is something neither of us could have imagined would ever happen.

I feel I am still making a difference to the lives of LGBT people. I'm learning a lot from working with sectors I'd not previously had much contact with and have talked at many of their events about my own experiences. Reflections offer examples of the challenges and successes encountered, and how to make changes. I was humbled and surprised to receive an honorary doctorate from the University of Exeter, having the privilege to attend the graduation ceremony with my wife by my side and address the congregation about my journey.

I smile to myself occasionally when I think that I now have a job where I say the words lesbian, gay, bisexual and trans out loud, nearly every day. Who would have thought?

And in spite of some of the low points I've experienced, I still have the envelope that my mum gave me as I boarded the train to join the Navy in 1986 … and it has remained unopened.

Chapter 10

To Serve, Love and Belong
Major Michael Brigham MBE
British Army, The Mercian Regiment

When I was 16 years old I had a secret that I thought nobody knew and surely no one would understand. If you've been reading this book then it will be no surprise that my secret was my sexual orientation. I was gay; I didn't feel ashamed, I didn't feel uncomfortable, but I really didn't understand why I was different. I knew I liked men and that most of my friends liked women, but I didn't understand why. I didn't know what to think. I was young and unsure of where these feelings had come from. There was one immutable consistency that I was sure of at 16: I was going to join the Army and my sexual orientation was never a consideration in that. I chose the Army, I never chose to be gay, but I wouldn't change either.

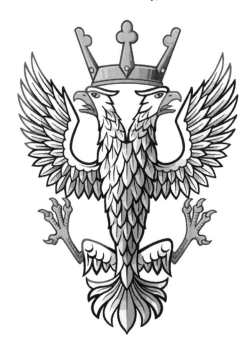

The Mercian regimental crest.

So there I was, 16 years old and certain of where I was going but not sure of who I was going to be when I got there. Finding who I would be, who I wanted to be and the journey I was about to start in the Armed Forces sets the context to my story, which I hope finds resonance with you, the reader.

I'm coming out, I want the world to know …

So everyone loves a good coming out story, but as often as they are humorous or heartwarming, they are dark or depressing. I, however, was blessed with a troubled upbringing in a loving home. We didn't have much, we were always on the breadline and life was hard, but my single-parent mother did the best she could. Looking back, I don't know why

I made such a fuss of telling my family that I was gay but I'm glad I told them when I did and that I didn't feel pressured to keep it a secret. So again, I find myself at 16 years old, walking into the small kitchen of the council house we occupied in Lyme Regis. It was early evening and the room was characteristically filled with cigarette smoke from my mother, who was washing up while daydreaming out of the kitchen window. My mum, Tracey, a proud Irish-Brummie, often daydreamed and I used to imagine she thought of herself on a small farm away from worries of debt and depression. I interrupted her thoughts by telling her I had something important to say. She turned, looked straight at me and said 'Make me a coffee' as she moved to sit at the kitchen table.

Coffee made, I sat next to her as she took a large gulp from her cup and said, 'Tell me.' Without hesitation I blurted out 'Mum, I'm gay,' and in return, also without hesitation, she jumped from the table, slapped me around the head and said, 'You bloody idiot. I thought you had someone pregnant. I don't care if you're gay; I just want you to be happy.' It was a massive anticlimax, with my brother and sister showing an equal lack of concern. Essentially, my moment, my coming-out swansong, was stolen by love; my nearest and dearest just didn't care about my sexual orientation.

It was 2001: it was legal to be gay in the Army; the fighting had been done and I was one of the lucky ones surrounded by those who just loved me for me. There was nothing stopping me answering that call to service.

Fast-forward six years and I was leaving Birmingham University Officer Training Corps and moving to 4 MERCIAN as a reserve officer. My time here was short; I was given a number of high profile roles within the reserves, one of which included training a platoon of reservist troops to deploy to Afghanistan with 2 MERCIAN, the regular unit I would later join. Many of the soldiers and officers in 4 MERCIAN were quite long in the tooth but I never met one who didn't like me because of my sexuality. The majority of the soldiers and officers I met quickly learnt to like and respect me because they were more interested in what I could do as a soldier rather than who I went to bed with at night. On leaving 4 MERCIAN I went through the regular Platoon Commanders' Battle Course and joined 2 MERCIAN.

***

Prior to my arrival in 2 MERCIAN it was known that a gay officer was going to arrive and that he was a cage fighter (taken out of context from my martial arts experience). I can honestly say I was more concerned that people would think I was overly aggressive than knowing I was gay, but nevertheless, both had me a little anxious. On arrival to 2 MERCIAN I was assigned to the support weapons company as the machine gun platoon commander. My immediate superior was the Officer Commanding of the support weapons company, Major, now Lieutenant

Colonel, Robert Moorhouse, known as Bob. As soon as I arrived, Bob sat me down and gave me his leadership guidance and at the end he said, 'So I know you're a homosexual and so does everyone else, but I'm not going to treat you any different and you shouldn't expect to act any different either.' It was delivered quite bluntly but it was the greatest gift he could have given me. He essentially told me that he had my back and to just be me. Until that point I was unsure how it was going to be in the Regular Army, but when I walked out I knew it was going to be OK. I integrated into the battalion without it being an issue. I'm sure there were some people who didn't like the fact I was gay but I have never had a single negative comment or action directed at me due to my sexuality. In contrast to harassment or difficulty, it actually at times created great amusement or laughter.

One such time was just prior to my first deployment to Afghanistan. A Welsh Guards officer called Major Robert Gallimore was attached to us for some pre-deployment training. In one of the evenings we were sat down playing cards and telling stories and he broached the subject about how at times the Army could be a little backward with some of its ways. He burst out, 'You know what we need? We need the first openly gay infantry officer. In actual fact, I would love to meet him and shake his hand when that happens.' Everyone burst out laughing and I walked over and extended my hand, saying, 'Hi Rob, that could be me.' Again the laughter roared as we went back to playing cards and telling stories.

There are numerous other times where my sexuality has caught people off guard. Normally it has been born from the manner in which I discuss my husband Danny. My method is simple: just don't think about it and make it natural, which inevitably means I use a variation of terms like 'partner', 'husband', 'he' or just his name. I used to have people correct me quite often by questioning if I had mistakenly said he rather than she and would find it amusing to say no, and anticipate their inevitable embarrassment. Another of my favourite surprise 'I'm gay' moments is the all too common expression of 'Oh' when I've literally had to spell it out after the person repeatedly says 'your wife' or 'what does she do?' etc. These moments are often followed by a demonstration of how many gay people they know and how they have no problem with me being gay. Sometimes, out of devilment, I reply that I also have no issue with them being straight.

Each of the circumstances described in my experience have been genuinely erroneous, with no malice, and have often led to shared laughter. In part I think I have a responsibility not to take offence to these situations, just as much as others should try to avoid them. I suspect these circumstances have occurred in the military due to me not conforming to stereotypes. In fact, if I fit into any stereotype, it's being a typical Army officer – one who dresses and dances just as badly as any other Army officer. It also doesn't help that my husband is a typical rugby lad from up north, who you wouldn't suspect was gay either. It isn't just the military that Danny and I catch off guard, and in all honesty, the general population is unintentionally more offensive, with statements like 'what a waste' or 'such a shame; my daughter would love you'. These circumstances are common to openly gay folks in all walks of life, but they are gradually diminishing.

One of the most important positive aspects of being openly gay in the British Army is fulfilling the requirement to be successful and effective role models for all personnel. I was incredibly fortunate as a young officer to have a more senior officer who was also gay in the unit, but he had not come out in the Army. He was a supporter of mine from day one and we are now very good friends. I remember one night at a regimental dinner he cornered me and said he was proud of me for being openly gay and asked whether I encountered any issues. I looked at him and told him that everyone knew he was gay; it was literally the worst kept secret in the regiment. He went straight over to his peers and came out to them, to which they replied that they had known for some time and gave him a bottle of champagne to open. He would tell you now that he was glad he had the courage to come out. He is currently a very open and comfortable senior gay role model in the British Army, whom I admire dearly.

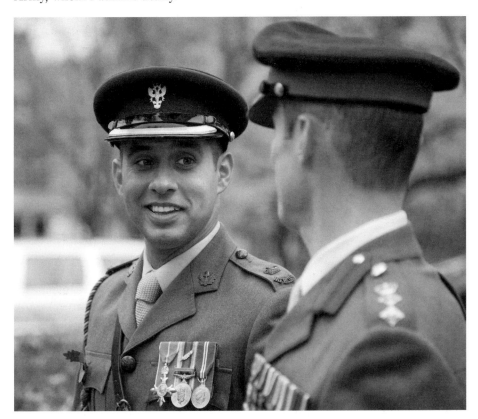

Remembrance Day, Fort Leavenworth. (*SemperFi Photography*)

The final part of this section and arguably the most important is how critical love is in the military. Not just love between soldiers, but also the love of those who support you. I can honestly say my husband is my key strength; he gives me energy, guides me when times are hard and provides a fundamental reason to keep our nation safe. Why would I want to keep that a secret, and how could I deny him being part of every aspect of my life? It was simple for me, but I understand that for others it may not be as easy.

The Army asks a lot from our loved ones and I never wanted Danny to have to face the sacrifice without the reward of the support network it affords. Never is that support network needed more than when we are on operations, and he has supported me through countless deployments. The first in Afghanistan was, without doubt, the hardest for him for many reasons, including the fact that we had only been together for just over a year.

***

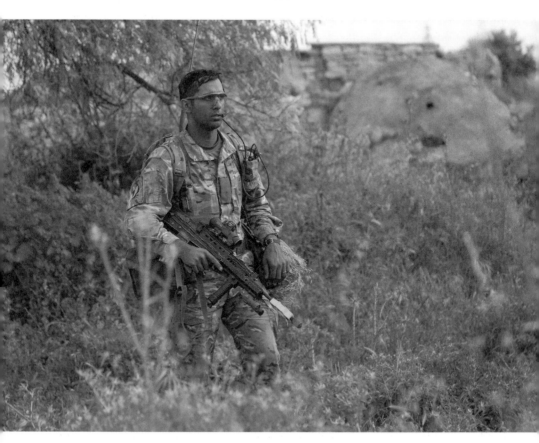

Training for operations, an apprenticeship in combat. (*SemperFi Photography*)

10 March 2009: ten days before my twenty-third birthday, I deployed on my first tour of Afghanistan as an operational mentor liaison team commander. It was the height of the conflict and an intense summer of fighting. Less than a year in battalion and I was getting ready to lead soldiers in close combat. Moreover, I was going to train the Afghan National Army (ANA) and have them fight alongside me. One thing was clear to me: bullets and improvised explosive devices (IEDs) don't discriminate. Needless to say, that summer in Afghanistan was incredibly challenging, with some life-changing events.

It made me a stronger person and a better Army officer, and also able to appreciate my loving partner. Further details of my exploits in Afghanistan can be read in Toby Harnden's *Dead Men Risen*, but there are three short stories that I wish to share with you here.

The first relates to my first month deployed – my combat apprenticeship. Prior to the deployment, I was paired with a platoon sergeant called Marc Giles, who was renowned for being as hard as coffin nails and a brilliant soldier. Sergeant Giles and I deployed ahead of our soldiers to the area we would assume responsibility for. We conducted our first familiarisation patrol on 17 March 2009. I was carrying some equipment that weighed what felt like a ton but provided protection to the team. Not long into the patrol we came under attack from the Taliban. It was ineffective small-arms fire from approximately 600 metres away but the first time you're shot at you don't know that. All you know is the drills you've been taught. I reacted as expected: no fault, no panic and no fear. I returned fire, took cover and observed, waiting to return fire at the enemy once the position was confirmed.

Marc Giles laughed at me and said, 'What you getting so excited for? You'll soon get used to this. Good job.' 'Good job' from Marc was huge praise and I remember feeling prouder in that instant than I had ever felt before.

In that moment I also realised that our soldiers' lives were at risk on every patrol we went on and that some might not come back if I didn't continue to do a good job. The first two weeks after my soldiers arrived I would go to Marc and ask what he thought we should do. The next two weeks I would go to him with a plan and he would inevitably ask had I thought of X, Y and Z, to which I would reply no, and work them into the plan. By the end of the first month he had stopped giving me his input and I was worried we had fallen out or drifted apart. I confronted him and again he laughed at me, saying, 'No, you madman, you've just got it now. I'll tell you when you're fucking up, sir, don't you worry.' I was now in command of my team; the experience I gained over that month was immeasurable and it was evident that the more seasoned soldiers respected me and looked to me as a leader they would follow, no matter how grave the situation. This for me is the first and most important lesson I learnt on operations: do the right thing 100 per cent, continue to listen, learn and take the experience of those around you.

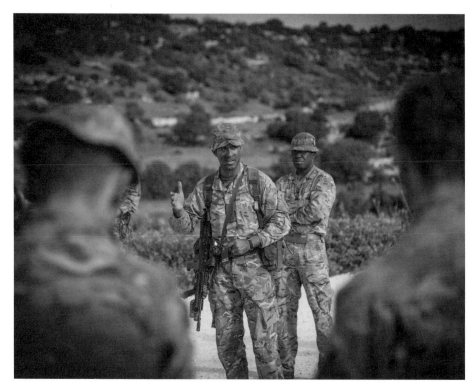

Briefing the teams before going on patrol – but I listened and learned and took experience from the whole team. (*SemperFi Photography*)

The second story relates to breaking down barriers. Around three months into my first tour of Afghanistan, a seasoned soldier, Colour Sergeant Ben Cox (Coxy) joined our team for a two-week period. He was assigned due to having not had much combat experience and wanting to get on the ground. Normally, my platoon sergeant and I would point-blank refuse to take 'combat tourists' on patrol with us because they were a liability, and frankly put our soldiers at risk. Coxy, however, was no liability; he was a machine. He was fit, robust and a fantastic soldier. If you were going to war, this is the man you would break out of the glass cage. I was honoured to have him with us. What I was not expecting was that Coxy was also a blooming bullet magnet.

On his first patrol with my team we were clearing a route and he found a suspected improvised explosive device (IED). As if that was not enough, we were shot at while he confirmed the IED and had to hold the position against the enemy force for seventy-two hours prior to the counter-IED team removing the device. The next fortnight continued in a similar manner. In two weeks he sure got his combat experience. I would guess he saw more action in that short period than most do in an entire career. It was time for Coxy to depart our team and return to his routine duties. We sat on the stairs of our patrol base accommodation and he turned to me and said, 'You know I'm from a pretty rough area, no Asians, and I didn't grow up with any gays, but you know what? You're alright.'

Now some might be outraged at this statement, but the reality is, you won't understand the bond of brotherhood and the openness and darkness of military humour until you have bled, sweated and cried with brother soldiers. The bond runs deep, deeper than I can explain in words, and as a result we speak freely and frankly. What Coxy was saying in his own way was that I'd changed his perspective, one that was probably entrenched from his social construction. He was telling me that he respected and loved me and that no matter what, he had my back. This was the second most important lesson I learnt on operations; the lesson is simple – context is king. Words, situations and actions out of context have no meaning, but in the light of context, sense can be made and meanings translated. This lesson helped me more than Coxy will ever know, and has continued to help me later in life.

The third story relates to the day that Marc Giles, my platoon sergeant, earned his Conspicuous Gallantry Cross (CGC), which is the second highest award for gallantry in the face of the enemy, second only to the Victoria Cross. It was 17 June 2009 and we deployed from our patrol base with the ANA. We totalled around forty troops – nine British and thirty-one ANA. We were tasked with clearing the enemy from a known stronghold and expected heavy Taliban resistance. It was part of the prelude to a major operation that would happen later that summer. As we set off on the patrol the ANA refused to progress along the given route, so I left my team and moved to the front of the patrol to personally lead the way. It was a calculated risk, designed to embarrass the ANA commander into progressing as planned.

I had a gut feeling that we should deviate from the route and cross a low wall over a field adjacent to a small mosque. This shortened our route by approximately 50 metres, but I would later realise that the gut feeling saved my life. As we progressed we came to a hedgerow that led to a tree line and was surrounded by three compounds. I knew it was highly likely we would be engaged as I moved into the open ground but knew this was the only way to root out the enemy and destroy this key stronghold.

As I progressed with the ANA we were immediately engaged by small-arms fire and bullets pierced my backpack. I returned fire and urged the soldier next to me to do the same, when he was shot, the bullet ripping through his hand and chest, killing him outright. There were approximately ten ANA and I caught in the open, pinned down by heavy enemy fire. I was the only one firing back until Marc Giles brought the British troops up and suppressed the enemy, no more than 200 metres from my location. I spoke to Marc on the radio and got him to move into cover, ordering a danger close airstrike to enable us to break from the position and gain an advantage over the enemy.

The airstrike came on the enemy position. I remember it clearly: a piercing sound, followed by a shockwave and a wall of dirt rushing over our position. It blinded the battlefield as dust and dirt lingered in the air, enabling Marc and I to collect the casualties and escape the killing area. We fought through the enemy position, clearing the stronghold and calling in another danger close airstrike to destroy enemy depth positions. The task was achieved and the battlefield was quiet.

As we withdrew with the two causalities, the enemy attacked us again. I commanded a rearguard action to create space between the enemy and our troops. Marc picked up both casualties and started to extract them under enemy fire, across open ground to a safe area. He was remarkable. We continued the rearguard for approximately 1,500 metres until we returned to the area of the mosque, where I had cut the corner over the low wall.

We occupied an area and called in support to extract the casualties. Approximately twenty-five minutes had passed and we were settled into routine when the enemy started to fire sporadically in our direction. This spooked the ANA and two of them ran towards the mosque, 5 metres beyond where I crossed the wall. Marc was not far behind. An IED detonated, throwing both the ANA and Marc into the air. Marc flew head first into a compound wall. I instantly checked if he was OK and he responded, 'Fuck off boss, I'm fine.' He ran forward with another soldier and began collecting the body parts of the ANA warriors who had been killed in the IED blast. The entire time he was under fire from the Taliban but he was focused on the mission and collected the warriors piece by piece.

I calmed the ANA and organised a defence of the location until an armoured vehicle patrol came and collected the casualties. We returned to our patrol base, debriefed the team and I wrote my report straight away. This patrol confirmed my belief that Marc is the bravest and best soldier I have ever known. That night I wrote Marc's citation and submitted it to my Officer Commanding (OC). When I got to bed, all I could think about was the ANA warriors who died in the IED by the mosque.

Six months after the tour, I was called by the Commanding Officer and was informed that Marc was to be awarded the CGC for his gallantry that day. I was so proud; he had earned it without doubt. The Commanding Officer also informed me that I was to be awarded a Queen's Commendation for Valuable Service (QCVS), represented by a silver oak leaf I wear upon my Afghanistan Medal. The citation for the QCVS reads:

> Acting Captain Brigham has led his Operational Mentoring and Liaison Team (OMLT) in Nad-e Ali and Basharan, both highly dangerous and kinetic operating areas. His team has mentored the Heavy Weapons Company of 1/3/205 Kandak Afghan National

Army (ANA). Brigham has emerged as the finest officer mentor in the OMLT Battlegroup, displaying professionalism, mental and physical robustness, and leadership of the highest standard on a daily basis.

Brigham has an intuitive grasp of mentoring; a role that requires enormous tact, patience, integrity and good judgement. Brigham's focus, drive and diligence has been an example to all. He encompassed all aspects of mentoring from Staff Branches S1 to S9 and continually looked to improve the ANA, without prompting. Brigham particularly emphasised to the ANA the benefits of influence and non-kinetic effects and as such he has been a driving force behind the genuine civil-military improvements taking place in Basharan. Without formal training he grasped the essentials of the Dari language and used it to his team's advantage. On operations and in social interaction with Afghan Warriors he has earned their respect and admiration in equal measure. Brigham immersed himself in Afghan culture in a way that is entirely respectful and without ever forgetting why he is there or allowing his standards as a British Army officer to slip.

Brigham has combined impressive mentoring with tactical acumen and bravery. He has repeatedly taken the lead in arduous combat operations and set an example that the ANA have tried to match. On 17 Jun 09, Brigham was mentoring a patrol of ANA to the south of Basharan. The patrol was in danger of falling apart before enemy contact began. The ANA refused repeatedly to progress along the agreed route and Brigham was forced to leave the safety of the Electronic Counter Measures bubble and prove personally that it was safe to continue. As Brigham led the way an ambush was initiated. Accurate and sustained small arms rained down and Rocket Propelled Grenade fire exploded among them from no more than 150 metres away. The Warriors immediately took cover, overwhelmed by the onslaught; Brigham stood his ground and was the only man standing and returning fire in an attempt to suppress the enemy. Unperturbed by the Warriors' reaction, he continued to engage and was under fire the entire time. An ANA Warrior was seriously wounded immediately next to him and Brigham's back pack pierced by bullets. The situation was so grave as he commanded the rear guard in a fighting withdrawal that he called for 2 danger close air strikes. Another Warrior was killed during the extraction by the explosion of an improvised explosive device, but Brigham was resolute under the pressure and inspired all around him.

Given his relative inexperience, his sublime mentorship, bravery, selfless dedication to the Afghan Warriors and inspirational leadership have been exemplary and far beyond what could have been expected. He deserves the highest formal public recognition.

To this day I don't know what made me cross that low wall and I never will. Perhaps it was God, but I'd heard he wouldn't love our sort. Perhaps it was luck, but I'd heard that to be gay isn't lucky. Maybe, just maybe, it was love. For in my life I was fortunate enough to know a god that loved me; to have the best of friends that only luck can provide; and have a love so strong that no matter how dark it gets, I'd always have a light to lead me home. And it did.

That love made me aware that luck was on my side and I believe it was God that made me cross that wall for no good reason – a wall that two of the Afghan National Army later ran past, leading to their deaths. From that moment, I have lived my life thankful for a feeling that made me survive that day, for the country that I serve and for those I hold dear to me.

***

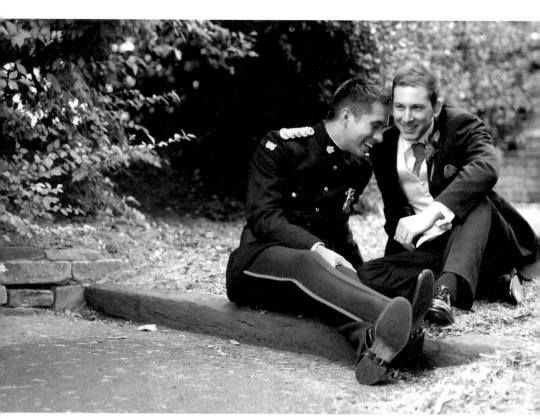

Danny and I on our wedding day. (*Lisa Carpenter Photography*)

Numerous other operational and training deployments furthered my experience and reputation. As time went on I continued to prove my worth, resulting in me promoting highly to Major in 2015. On promotion I was selected to attend the United States Command and General Staff College (CGSC) and was given an opportunity to attend selection for a second year at the most prestigious United States School of Advanced Military Studies (SAMS), colloquially known as the 'book a night, Jedi planners' course'. Needless to say, I was successful in the selection and performed very well at both CGSC and SAMS. I was fully prepared for the USA and for life as an openly gay couple on a US military base to be a little different from what it was in the UK. My husband and I had a simple approach to handle this: don't change, don't hide, do what we've always done and be happy with being us.

Now I know you are expecting that Danny and I faced a torrent of abuse and homophobic behaviour while in the United States but in fact it was quite the opposite. When we first got there we had the routine shock and surprise effect that we have on everyone – how could two normal guys be gay and happily married? My favourite reaction that routinely occurred in the US was when someone met me first and subsequently met Danny. They often built an impression in their minds that Danny would be an effeminate male and were quite shocked to meet a good rugby lad from northern England. This caused us no end of amusement and delightfully awkward situations that often led to good friendships.

As time went on we built more friendships in the USA. By our second year everyone knew us, or at least knew who we were, and more importantly, knew we threw the best dinner parties and events. Without realising, we had become positive role models who had made quite an impact in the community. On numerous occasions we had complete strangers come up to us and thank us for being so open, as it had enabled them to understand and deal with homosexuality in their own lives. Twice we directly counselled senior military officers about their teenage or adult children, which enabled them to repair relationships. In one such case, we have remained close friends with a couple who are now enjoying catching up on years of lost time with their beloved son.

At the end of our time in the USA, Danny and I were awarded a commendation by the Defence Attaché for our community engagement and efforts to be positive role models. A very senior British general spoke to Danny and me at a baseball game and asked if anything was different being a same-sex couple on a US military base compared to being in the UK. I responded by saying, 'Well the main difference is that in the UK, you and I wouldn't be having this conversation as it's really a non-issue in our army, but in the USA you feel the need to ensure I am OK.' We both laughed.

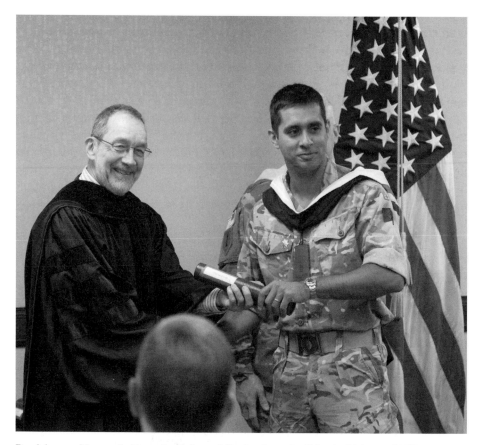

Receiving my Masters in Operational Art and Design from the School of Advanced Military Studies in Fort Leavenworth, Kansas.

***

When I mentioned to the General that I believed homosexuality in the British Army is a non-issue, I sincerely meant it. I know this is not a popular statement but to my mind it is an accurate one. I was the lead for the first army-led LGBT conference at the time that Respect for Others was published. For me this was a milestone in the British Army. The Respect for Others policy is simple: everyone gets treated the same and gets treated with respect. It also coincided with the change in the Army's policy for same-sex couples being recognised with the same status as heterosexual couples. Ever since this policy change, the practices have only improved. We have the processes to ensure the policies are implemented, and moreover, we have the process to ensure that breaches in policy are rectified.

What the Army now needs is less flag-waving and more confidence. We don't have to fight for LGBT rights in the Army anymore; we need to have confidence to do our jobs knowing the system protects us. The youngest soldiers that join the Army are supportive and accepting of the LGBT community. This became apparent to me when I assumed command of my infantry company and a new soldier joined from training. The soldier asked if I was married and I said yes, to my husband Danny. He didn't even blink, just carried on, and asked where he was from and what he did. To me this reinforced my perspective that those who had come before me had done the fighting on my behalf. They had made my life in the Army easy. I just needed to be the best I could be and have confidence in the system.

***

I told you at the start of my story that I was always destined to become a soldier. When I was younger it was about the thrill, the adventure and the opportunity to make a better life for myself. As time goes on my service has become much more altruistic: I genuinely believe the only thing that allows evil to succeed is good men doing nothing.

I also believe that the Armed Forces are a fantastic employer, enabling social mobility and delivering life experiences beyond measure. I am blessed in my life by three things: the love of friends and family; the love of my husband and his love returned; and love for the British Army. I am lucky to have a career that promotes my success, irrespective of the colour of my skin or my sexual orientation. And an employer that strives for equality and inclusivity … and that gives me more than a job: it provides me with a calling, and a destiny, which I'm proud to call mine.

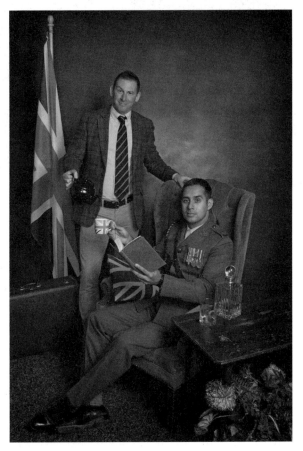

A love so strong I'd always have a light to lead me home.

Glossary

2IC	Second-in-command
AAC	Army Air Corps
AIB	Admiralty Interview Board
AIDS	Acquired immune deficiency syndrome
ANA	Afghanistan National Army
ARF	Airborne Reaction Force
AZT	Zidovudine (anti-HIV drug)
BSA	Bosnian Serb Army
BNF	British National Formulary
BRNC	Britannia Royal Naval College
CGC	Conspicuous Gallantry Cross
CGRM	Command General Royal Marines
CGSC	Command and General Staff College
CHF	Commando Helicopter Force (RN)
CMH	Cambridge Military Hospital (Aldershot)
CN	Counternarcotics
CND	Campaign for Nuclear Disarmament
CO	Commanding Officer
CW	Commissioning warrant
COMCLYDENORLANT	Commodore Clyde and North Atlantic
D&I	Diversity & Inclusion
dit	military term for a story or yarn
ECHR	European Convention on Human Rights / European Court of Human Rights
E&D	Equality & Diversity
EDA	European Defence Agency
EOD	Explosives Ordnance Team
GCHQ	Government Communications Headquarters
GI	Gunnery Instructor
HADR	Humanitarian Assistance and Disaster Relief
HIV	Human Immunodeficiency Virus
HMG	Her Majesty's Government
HPAT	Homosexuality Policy Assessment Team
HR	Human Resources
HTIC	Helicopter Tactics Instructor Course

IED	Improvised Explosive Device
IFOR	Implementation Force (NATO)
JHC	Joint Helicopter Command
LGB	Lesbian, gay, bisexual
LGBT	Lesbian, gay, bisexual and transgender
LGBTQ	Lesbian, gay, bisexual, transgender, queer or questioning
MANPADS	Man-portable air-defence system
MBE	Member of the Most Excellent Order of the British Empire
MIRT	Medical Immediate Response Team
MoD	Ministry of Defence
NAAFI	Navy, Army and Air Force Institutes
NATO	North Atlantic Treaty Organisation
OMLT	Operational Mentor and Liaison Team
Pl Comd	Platoon Commander
Pl Sgt	Platoon Sergeant
PSO	Personal Selection Officer
PWO	Principal Warfare Officer
OC	Officer Commanding
OM	Order of Merit
OST	Operational sea training
QA/QARANC	Queen Alexandra's Royal Army Nursing Corps
QCVS	Queen's Commendation for Valuable Service
OTs	Overseas Territories
REME	Royal Electrical and Mechanical Engineers
RGN	Registered General Nurse
RNLI	Royal National Lifeboat Institution
RWOETU	Rotary Wing Operational Evaluation and Training Unit
SAMS	School of Advanced Military Studies
SIB	Special Investigation Branch
SOO(SA)	Staff Operations Officer (Surface and Air)
SOO(SM)	Staff Operations Officer Submarines
SOS	Special Operations Squadron
SSAFA	the Armed Forces charity (formerly, the Soldiers, Sailors, Airmen and Families Association)
UN	United Nations
URNU	University Royal Naval Unit
USN	United States Navy
VO	Vetting officer

WIGS	West Indies Guard Ship
WO	Warrant Officer
WRAC	Women's Royal Army Corps
WRNS	Women's Royal Naval Service
XO	Executive Officer